Exactly the kind of practical, thoughtful advice parents need when seeking treatment for their child's emotional, behavioral, or developmental disorders. I strongly recommend this book not only for parents but also for educators and pediatricians.
—*Bruce Masek, PhD, Associate Professor of Psychology, Harvard Medical School, Boston, MA*

Finally parents can learn what science has to say about child mental health problems and the ways to most effectively treat these problems. This clear and highly readable book contains the facts, not the fiction—allowing parents to be successful in accomplishing the task in the title.
—*Wendy Silverman, PhD, ABPP, Professor of Psychology, Florida International University, Miami*

In this compassionate and readable book, Braaten guides parents through the difficult process of finding appropriate mental health care for the child who is struggling. Parents will find practical advice tempered with the thoughtfulness and understanding that comes from years of helping children and the parents who love them. I highly recommend this book.
—*Michael A. Tompkins, PhD, Assistant Clinical Professor, University of California, Berkeley; author of* My Anxious Mind: A Teen's Guide to Managing Anxiety and Panic

How *to* Find
Mental Health Care
for
Your Child

How *to* Find Mental Health Care *for* Your Child

Ellen B. Braaten, PhD

American Psychological Association • *Washington, DC*

Published by
APA Lifetools
750 First Street, NE
Washington, DC 20002
www.apa.org

To order
APA Order Department
P.O. Box 92984
Washington, DC 20090-2984
Tel: (800) 374-2721;
Direct: (202) 336-5510
Fax: (202) 336-5502;
TDD/TTY: (202) 336-6123
Online: www.apa.org/pubs/books/
E-mail: order@apa.org

In the U.K., Europe, Africa, and the Middle East, copies may be ordered from
American Psychological Association
3 Henrietta Street
Covent Garden, London
WC2E 8LU England

Typeset in Sabon by Circle Graphics, Columbia, MD

Printer: United Book Press, Baltimore, MD
Cover Designer: Naylor Design, Washington, DC

The opinions and statements published are the responsibility of the authors, and such opinions and statements do not necessarily represent the policies of the American Psychological Association.

Library of Congress Cataloging-in-Publication Data
Braaten, Ellen.
  How to find mental health care for your child / Ellen B. Braaten.
    p. cm.
  Includes bibliographical references and index.
  ISBN-13: 978-1-4338-0898-2
  ISBN-10: 1-4338-0898-6
  ISBN-13: 978-1-4338-0899-9 (e-book)
  ISBN-10: 1-4338-0899-4 (e-book)
  1. Child mental health services—Popular works. 2. Child psychiatry—Popular works. I. Title.

  RJ499.34.B73 2011
  362.198'9289—dc22
                                   2010020485

British Library Cataloguing-in-Publication Data
A CIP record is available from the British Library.

Printed in the United States of America
First Edition

For my Mom, Roberta,
and my daughter, Hannah.
Thank you for
teaching me everything
I have needed to know.

CONTENTS

How *to* Find
Mental Health Care
for
Your Child

INTRODUCTION

As a child psychologist who evaluates hundreds of children each year, I have the honor of guiding parents through the difficult process of coming to a clearer understanding of their child's strengths and weaknesses. Many times, parents arrive at my office distraught over issues such as their child's lack of academic progress, difficulty in forming friendships, problems with hyperactivity or focus, or trouble regulating mood or behavior. In my experience, I have rarely found that parents incorrectly identify their children's need for help, but frequently parents have spent months trying to figure out what their child needs and how to get the right kind of help. For example, Sarah was a 12-year-old girl who never had difficulties with attention until the past year, after watching her parents go through a very messy divorce. Her parents wondered if problems in school were the result of an undiagnosed learning disability, familial stress, or anxiety, but they did not know where to turn. Carl's parents on the other hand, wondered why Carl, their 8-year-old son, wasn't reading. Carl's teacher told them not to worry; they knew something was wrong and wanted to know why, but they had no idea who could best answer their questions or where to turn.

These parents are not alone; it is estimated that between 12% and 24% of American children suffer from psychological disorders at some point in their development. Parents whose children struggle with issues such as depression, anxiety, learning disorders, and attention problems face tough questions such as, Does my child need medication? Does my child have a learning disability? How do I get an appropriate diagnosis? How can I ensure that my child gets the best possible treatment? What do I need to know to monitor my child's care and find the most competent professional?

In my work with parents, I have found that seeking mental health care is one of the most anxiety-provoking decisions that many parents face, largely because they don't know where to go and what to expect once they get there. Many (or perhaps most) parents don't know the difference between a psychologist, psychiatrist, or social worker. They are baffled when confronted with terms such as *cognitive behavior therapy, neuropsychological evaluation,* and *mood dysregulation.* In addition, they don't merely want to be told to "get a prescription"; they want to understand what their child's underlying condition is and what causes it. They want to know what treatments are available and how helpful each of them might be. Above all they want hope that their child will get better.

The purpose of this book is to anticipate and answer the questions parents might have when they are confronted with a child who is struggling. Although there are a number of books that have explored specific issues, such as how to parent a child who has attention-deficit/hyperactivity disorder or Asperger's disorder or is depressed or explosive, in this book, I help parents who do not know what to do when their child develops problems. I discuss what the psychological literature has to say about the symptoms and types of mental health illnesses that children can develop as well as the types of therapies, therapists, and treatments available to them. I address concerns that arise when parents are just beginning to worry about what could be wrong and what they can do about it. I discuss what parents in real situations did when confronted with problems and provide the full variety of treatments that have been shown to be effective for particular problems. Most important, it is my hope that this book will provide reassurance, encouragement, and general support for parents along the sometimes stressful journey of parenting by empowering them with the most important tool of all—information.

In Part I: What Every Parent Should Know About Child Psychology and Mental Health Disorders, I provide an overview of the issues involved in diagnosing and treating psychological disorders. I present common concerns that parents might have and provide information about normal child development so that parents can determine whether their child's issues fall within the normal range. In Part I, I also provide information about the diagnostic process and treatment possibilities. In Chapter 1, I present an overview of the types of problematic behaviors that children may exhibit at different times in development and provide background in helping parents decide whether to go ahead and have their child evaluated for possible treatment. In Chapter 2, I provide general guidelines as to when to seek help, the elements of different types of evaluations, and what to look for in a competent professional. I review the possible choices parents have (e.g., psychiatric evaluation, consultation with a psychologist, neuropsychological testing, meeting with the school psychologist) and explain the positive and possible negatives of each possibility. In Chapter 3, I help orient parents to the possible treatments that are available within psychology and psychiatry. This chapter includes explanations of terms such as *cognitive behavior therapy, psychodynamic therapy, family therapy,* and *play therapy.* School-based, clinic-based, and hospital-based treatments are reviewed.

In Part II: Common Childhood Disorders, I provide information about common symptoms, biology, causes, course (i.e., what happens to a child with this disorder over time), and treatment options for the major psychological and learning disorders that are seen in children and adolescents. In each chapter, I discuss the best treatment options and where to seek each type of treatment (e.g., hospital, school, licensed psychologist, psychiatrist). Disorders include attention-deficit/ hyperactivity disorder, autism and pervasive developmental disorders, mood disorders such as depression and bipolar disorder, anxiety disorders, learning disabilities, and eating disorders.

In Part III: The Treatments, I review detailed information on the treatments referred to in Parts I and II—how therapists think the treatments work, which disorders they are used to treat, the typical course of treatment, and what to look for to determine whether the treatment is effective. Treatments include insight-oriented therapies; play therapy; cognitive behavior therapy; family therapy; school-based services; and allied treatments such as medication, occupational therapy, and speech therapy. Finally, the book includes resources that provide an annotated list of organizations that promote mental health in children and adolescents as well as books and websites for particular disorders.

You may not read this book from cover-to-cover, although it might be helpful to read Part I and then read the chapters that focus more on your child's diagnostic or treatment needs. In contrast, you might find yourself reading the book straight through because it can inform you about issues that you had never thought of. One thing to consider is that it is quite common for psychological disorders to coexist; in other words, many children have more than one disorder. Furthermore, it is quite common for treating professionals to use more than one approach—a psychologist may use techniques from cognitive behavior therapy along with play therapy, or a child may receive school-based services and medication. The combinations of treatment approaches are endless. Thus, it is quite likely that if you have sought treatment, more that one chapter in Part III may apply to you.

This book won't answer all your questions, nor will it enable you to determine your child's exact diagnosis or best treatment. It may help you along this process by providing you with information to ask the right questions while helping you better understand the process. The resources at the end of the book provide helpful information about where to go from here. Above all, know that you are not alone in this process. It is my hope that this book may help you and your child find the help you need. Finally, this book is filled with examples from my clinical practice. These cases are composites of actual cases and are not real patients. Clinical situations have been disguised in a number of ways to protect patient confidentiality, and no child's real name or information was used.

Part I

WHAT EVERY PARENT SHOULD KNOW ABOUT CHILD PSYCHOLOGY AND MENTAL HEALTH DISORDERS

CHAPTER I

DOES MY CHILD HAVE A PROBLEM?

Parenting is fraught with anxiety, and caring parents want desperately to "do the right thing." It is never easy for parents to consider the possibility that their child might have a mental, emotional, learning, or behavioral problem. Most parents know little about the subject of psychological and learning disorders and even less about treatment. This lack of knowledge can leave parents feeling plagued with guilt that they may have "done something wrong" and worrying about what it might mean for their child's future.

Guilt and confusion were readily apparent when I first met David's parents. They told me that David had always seemed like a bright child. From an early age, he would take apart things such as the radio or phone, hoping to figure out how they worked. They thought this was a sign of intellect and curiosity; others in the family thought he was just "getting into everything." Although he was a bit late to talk, once he started, he never stopped talking. His parents took his hyperactivity and eccentricities in stride until they received a call from the kindergarten teacher telling them she was concerned that David could not focus and was disruptive to the other children. The teacher recommended consulting with a professional about his behavior, but his parents fretted for months about whom to call first (psychologist? psychiatrist? pediatrician?) and what the problem could be.

Leslie's parents thought their 16-year-old seemed to have the whole world ahead of her, so they were confused as to why she was spending so much time in her room. She had gotten stellar grades until her parents separated last year, but since then has seemed quiet and sad. Now her grades are suffering, and college applications are not far away. Leslie's parents know she needs help, but they aren't sure if their daughter's behavior is serious or just normal for a teenager.

How common are problems such as Leslie's and David's? Well, it's difficult to say because the line between normal and abnormal behavior is often a matter of degree. That said, most children show at least some kind of problem behavior at one time or another. Best estimates are that about one child in five has an actual mental health problem that significantly impairs function, and 10% to 20% of children meet diagnostic criteria for a specific psychological disorder. Many other children have mild problems or adjustment difficulties, such as adjusting to a new school or family situation, that may make them behave in ways that are inappropriate for their age. Determining which problems merit professional attention and which ones don't is difficult and in many ways depends on the degree to which the problem is interfering with the child's functioning. Often parents know instinctively that something is not right, only to be told by friends, family members, and even professionals such as doctors and teachers that there is nothing to worry about. Other times, friends and family will remark how Johnny seems to have a problem, but parents are not ready to hear it. Usually, though, professionals label a child's behaviors as problematic if the problem persists for more than 3 or 4 weeks without going away or if the problem is at the end of the continuum for that behavior. Another consideration is whether the symptoms are appropriate for the age of the child. For example, a 5-year-old child might start wetting the bed after her family moves to a new town. This would be considered inappropriate but somewhat normal under the circumstances (especially if the behaviors last only a week or so), whereas a 9-year-old who displays the same behaviors, which do not remit after a few weeks, for example, would be considered worthy of an evaluation.

IS THIS SOMETHING TO BE WORRIED ABOUT?

Psychological problems are much more prevalent than most parents realize. Many experts in the field of child psychology agree that there are two main categories of problematic disorders: *externalizing problems* in which the behavior is expressed outward through hyperactivity, aggression, defiance, bullying, or delinquency; and *internalizing problems* in which the problematic behavior is directed inward or internally, as is the case with depression, anxiety, and eating disorders. An additional area of concern relates to the field of *learning disabilities;* these problems are neither externalizing nor internalizing but relate to a child's ability to progress academically at a pace commensurate with his or her peers. Furthermore, many emotional and behavior disorders tend to overlap with other disabilities, such as learning disabilities.

In terms of defining significant problems that are worthy of professional attention, the following guidelines might be helpful:

- *Behavior that is extreme*—such behavior is not just a bit different or "off" but very different from that of one's peers or severe in intensity.
- *Problems that are chronic*—these problems either never go away (such as daily temper tantrums or constant sadness) or keep reappearing (such as anxiety that is intense for a few weeks, goes away, but comes back again).

- *Multiple symptoms*—these are symptoms that may not seem very serious by themselves, but in combination they can be alarming, such as difficulty concentrating, poor self-esteem, and problems learning to read.
- *Significant consequences*—these include behaviors that are extremely serious, such as an expulsion from school or truancy, a suicide attempt, or problems with alcohol or drugs. Even though these behaviors may not be chronic (i.e., may not have occurred for months), their significance indicates they warrant immediate attention.
- *Failure to progress at a rate similar to peers*—in the early years this can include behaviors such as language skills or social skills that are not developing on time, whereas in the elementary school years this can include skills such as reading or writing.

Understanding whether a child's problem needs the attention of a professional begins with gaining knowledge about child development and the norms of behavioral problems. Being a well-informed parent is vital, especially when knowing what to expect from one's child at different ages can be the key to understanding whether his or her behavior is normal. But many parents discover that figuring out what to expect of their children at different ages can be very challenging. Parents who have more than one child always seem to be surprised how very different their children can be—yet each child would be considered "normal." Some of the more significant causes for concern are listed on page 16, but many of these symptoms are fairly common behaviors that occur to some extent in all children (in fact you may notice some in yourself!); for example, difficulty completing schoolwork, problems concentrating, and feelings of sadness are things everyone may have experienced at one time or another. It is the *intensity, frequency,* and *severity* of the behaviors that determine whether the problems warrant further attention. The information in Part II of this book is provided to help you understand whether your child's symptoms meet the criteria for seeking professional help, but keep in mind that although understanding the particular symptoms are important, it is just as important to understand that these symptoms need to be severe enough and to occur at such a frequency that they impact the child's ability to function at an age-appropriate level.

In general, problems with mood, such as anxiety, panic, and depression, are common reasons to seek a mental health consultation. It can be difficult for parents who are not experiencing these symptoms to determine whether their child is depressed because children's symptoms of depression and anxiety do not always look like those one sees in adults. Children do not necessarily articulate their nervousness or appear to be sad but may instead be irritable or even hostile. They may be tired, have trouble sleeping, or lose interest in things they used to enjoy. Other common reasons for a consultation include problems making and keeping friends or an inability to build or maintain satisfactory relationships with peers; an inability to perform in school; problems with concentration or hyperactivity; or conduct problems such as truancy, theft, frequent underage drinking or illegal drug use.

NOW THAT I KNOW I SHOULD BE WORRIED, WHAT SHOULD I DO FIRST?

If you've picked up this book, it is very likely that you have given some thought to the idea that your child might have a problem. Very often, the first person to consult is your child's pediatrician—this is especially true if your child is not yet in elementary school. Once children reach school age, the teacher or school guidance counselor is often the first person you may want to consult. In the case of consulting with your child's pediatrician, it is wise to have thought

Possible Causes for Concern

Concern is warranted if the following behaviors are significantly interfering with a child's ability to function appropriately in school, at home, or with friends and if the symptoms are chronic, frequent, and don't remit after a few weeks:

- problems concentrating or paying attention in the school and home environments;
- temper tantrums that increase in intensity and frequency;
- difficulty following directions;
- uncooperativeness to the point of interfering with family or school functioning;
- problems completing homework on a regular basis;
- difficulty learning to read, spell, write, or complete schoolwork;
- truancy from school or frequent detentions or expulsions;
- chronically lacking in self-confidence or chronic feelings of worthlessness or feeling inferior to peers;
- feelings of sadness, depression, or anxiety that last more than 2 weeks and chronic feelings of self-consciousness, hypersensitivity, and fearfulness that never go away;
- problems mastering developmental norms on time, including things such as toilet training, social relationships, and language development; and
- showing bizarre behavior such as far-fetched ideas, repetitive speech, mania, or psychosis (seeing or hearing things that are not there).

a bit about what is most troubling about your child's behavior before mentioning your concerns. This will help the doctor focus on evaluating the exact issues that are troubling you, while helping to point you in the right direction. Pediatricians can help you decide whether you should have a referral to a psychologist, psychiatrist, or another type of therapist (such as an occupational or speech therapist). It is unlikely that your pediatrician will diagnose the problem in the office; instead, he or she will make a quick assessment of the problem behaviors and help you figure out the next step you need to take. This might mean a referral to a psychiatrist for a medication evaluation, to a psychologist or social worker for psychotherapy, or to a neuro-psychologist or school psychologist for an evaluation. At times, the pediatrician might tell you to "wait and see," and often this is the right approach. Sometimes it isn't. I mentioned earlier that "trusting your gut" is an important cue, and it's important enough to reiterate here. If you are awake at night worrying about a particular problem and your doctor, partner, or neighbors say "don't worry"—but the worries just won't go away—it's probably time to get more information and consider a second opinion. It is possible that there really is nothing to worry about, but it is also likely you need more information and a referral to a specialist for a consult.

There are a few ways to approach seeking information from the school. If your child is 3 years of age or younger, you can seek help by accessing the early intervention services in your local county or school district. They can provide free assessments that evaluate a child's psychological and development needs. Once a child is in school and when you sense something is not right, it can be helpful to contact the teacher to see if she is seeing any of the same symptoms you are observing at home. For example, Brian seemed anxious and frequently washed his hands at home, and his mom was worried his nervousness and hand washing were becoming more than just a habit. She placed a call to Brian's teacher to ask him if he observed any of the same problems. When he admitted that he was worried, too, Brian's mom decided to call her pediatrician to get a referral to a child psychologist who could more thoroughly evaluate these issues. In the meantime, Brian's teacher suggested that Brian meet with the school psychologist because Brian seemed to be having difficulties getting along with his peers and frequently looked stressed.

The selection of a practitioner depends somewhat on the presenting problem. This book focuses primarily on treatments provided by clinical psychologists, although it should be noted that many other types of professionals are well qualified to administer treatments as well. Psychologists typically have a PhD (a doctorate of philosophy) or PsyD (a doctorate of psychology). Both have similar training as it relates to treating and evaluating patients. Doctoral-level psychologists spend at least 4 years (after completing college) training in the assessment and treatment of psychological disorders. In addition, they complete a full-time year-long internship followed by a year's worth of supervised postdoctoral training. Because this book relates to childhood disorders, the professionals who treat these disorders are typically *child psychologists* who have specialized in treating children and families. Some child psychologists also specialize in psychological testing; others specialize in particular types of therapies such as cognitive behavior therapy or family therapy. You will want to know that the psychologist you consult with has expertise in the area that you need. Information in Parts II and III of this book can help you determine what type of problem and what type of treatment (and specialist) you might need.

In addition to (or sometimes instead of) child psychologists, there are other professionals you might like to consult. They might include *neuropsychologists,* who are typically clinical psychologists who specialize in using neuropsychological tests to evaluate intellectual, memory, language, and visual–motor skills (among others) to diagnose problems such as learning disabilities, attention problems, and developmental disorders. It is probably no surprise to hear that *school psychologists* typically work in the school setting, where they frequently counsel students and administer tests. *Child psychiatrists* are physicians who specialize in the treatment of psychological and psychiatric disorders in children. Psychiatrists, because they are medical doctors, can prescribe medication, whereas psychologists cannot in most states. Other professionals include *speech and language therapists* (who evaluate and treat speech and language disorders), *occupational therapists* (who evaluate and treat issues such as fine motor and sensory integration difficulties), and *physical therapists* (who evaluate and treat gross motor and physical functioning). Child psychologists are typically well versed in the types of services that other professionals provide and may make recommendations to professionals such as these.

WHAT IF WE JUST WAIT AND SEE?

There's nothing wrong with just waiting and watching, if that is what feels right for you. In fact, it is often initially the best course of action. To wait and see is actually not doing nothing, particularly if you are monitoring and observing your child's symptoms. While you are observing, it can also be a good time to get more information—talk to friends and relatives, gather more information, and watch to make sure that the symptoms are not getting worse. A good general rule of thumb is to be more proactive the older your child is. For example, if a child is struggling in school in kindergarten, it might be best to wait until first grade before evaluating what could be causing the problem, but waiting a full year to see if your eighth grader (who is all of a sudden getting poor grades) gets better might be too long to wait. That being said, there is a wealth of data that show the importance of intervening early, and thus, if your child has been diagnosed with a problem, make sure he is she is getting the best treatment possible.

Thus, although waiting is sometimes the right course of action, in my experience parents often wish they had not waited quite so long to seek treatment. If you are one of those parents, don't fret over the time lost. Every good parent feels guilty about something, but it's usually not a very useful emotion. In fact, child psychologists frequently miss symptoms in their own children and wish they had sought help sooner, and they do this for a living! It's never too late to find the right treatment, and gathering information (as you are doing by reading this book) is an important first step. In Chapter 2, I describe the first step you will encounter when seeking help: the evaluation.

What to Do When You're Worried Your Child Is Too Much Like You or Someone Else in the Family

It can be discouraging for many parents who struggled for years to overcome their own issues of anxiety, depression, or learning disabilities only to find similar issues in their child. It can be frightening if a father observed his own mother experience bouts of depression and common for him to worry that a diagnosis of depression in his daughter will mean that his child will turn out "just like Grandma." I frequently counsel parents not to assume it will be the same for their child as it might have been for them or another family member. Remember: Biology is not destiny. Furthermore, most of us (and particularly our parents) grew up in a time when little was known about psychological disorders. Many people who needed services never got the diagnosis they needed, and if they did, the treatments were few and possibly unsubstantiated. Although there is more to be researched and discovered, we know vastly more about childhood mental health and disorders than we did a generation ago. With the right treatment, even if a child's depression does seem just like Grandma's, the course of the depression can be dramatically different from Grandma's as a result of treatments that unfortunately were not available in the past.

In my experience, parents in this situation often fall into two camps: They either tend to ignore the problem (until it's too late) or become overly anxious (long before they need to or at an intensity that is unwarranted on the basis of the facts). Neither of these reactions is beneficial. The best course of action is to know your family's genetic history without over-analyzing or overreacting to every possible problem and to seek a consultation when you have significant concerns that do not go away.

CONCLUDING THOUGHTS

Psychological problems in childhood are more common that many people realize, and the types of problems and causes are quite varied. In this chapter, I have provided a very brief overview of some of the more common problems that are seen in children and adolescents, but if you are worried about your child and his or her problem is not on this list, definitely seek help. Your child's pediatrician and school personnel are good places to start, and there are other professionals, such as clinical psychologists and psychiatrists, who can further evaluate any concerns as necessary.

CHAPTER 2

THE EVALUATION:
FINDING OUT WHAT IS WRONG

Once parents have decided to seek an evaluation or treatment for
their child, the array of choices can be confusing. Each of the professional disciplines mentioned in Chapter 1 has pros and cons, and
your selection should be guided in a large part by the type of problem your child is exhibiting. In reality, however, the professional
whom you ultimately see may be determined by your insurance coverage and the types of mental health services available where you
live. You also may not know the best person to contact until after
you have had an initial appointment with a professional. This may
be the person who will then help you find the best professional for
your child's particular problem. Luckily, there is significant overlap
between professionals.

GUIDELINES FOR HANDLING YOUR CHILD'S PROBLEMS

Here are some general guidelines to knowing who the best specialist is for your child's particular problem and what to do in various
circumstances. Most important, though, any of the professionals
mentioned in the paragraphs that follow need to have specialized
training and experience with children and adolescents.

The Problem Is New, and There Has Never Been Any Type of Diagnosis

If your child has recently exhibited a new, significant problematic behavior, you will need a professional who is skilled in diagnosing disorders. In this case, a child psychologist or a child psychiatrist is your best option. Child psychologists and psychiatrists are trained in interviewing and diagnosing, but simply consulting with them does not mean they will actually make a diagnosis. In fact, they may tell you that your child's problem is not a problem at all, or conversely, they may refer you to a different, more specialized therapist.

You Think Your Child May Need Medication

If you already suspect that your child needs medication for an attention problem, anxiety, or depression, you will need to consult a medical doctor. Most child psychiatrists prescribe medications, although a few of them practice only psychotherapy. Pediatricians also prescribe medications and can be a useful resource, particularly if you child's problem is relatively uncomplicated. Although nurse practitioners and physician assistants can prescribe medications, most often you would first want to consult with a medical doctor who could make a diagnosis and then refer to you a nurse practitioner or physician assistant to monitor your treatment.

> Professionals who can prescribe medications include medical doctors such as pediatricians, child psychiatrists, family practitioners, primary care physicians, and pediatric neurologists; doctors of osteopathy; nurse practitioners; and physician assistants.

You Think Your Child May Need Therapy

In this case, you will have many professionals from whom to

choose. These can include psychologists, psychiatrists, social workers, licensed professional counselors, and family therapists. Any of these professionals can have specialized training treating your child's particular disorder; the important issues are that the professional's area of specialty is a good match for your child and the professional is sufficiently experienced.

You Think Your Family May Need Therapy

Sometimes, the problem is not with one particular child but with the family system itself. For example, the family might have experienced a loss or significant stress, or perhaps family members are having trouble getting along, and the entire family would benefit from treatment. In this case, you would want to consult with a person who has specialized training in family therapy. Some states have particular licenses for marriage and family therapists, but many psychologists, psychiatrists, or social workers also specialize in this area as well.

Your Child's Problem Is Primarily Related to School Performance

If your child is having academic difficulties in school, the contact person of choice would be either your child's school psychologist, a pediatric neuropsychologist, or a child psychologist who specializes in psychological and neuropsychological assessment. Typically, if problems in this area involve learning, attentional, or motivational issues, testing will need to be performed. This can be done within the school system or outside of the school system. Sometimes parents will do a combination approach with some of the testing done at school and other aspects of the evaluation completed by a psychologist outside of the school system. However, you should note that schools do not typically diagnose children; they use testing to describe the behaviors and to make recommendations for school programming. If getting a firm diagnosis is important to you (such as knowing whether your child's symptoms are the result of dyslexia or attention-deficit/hyperactivity disorder [ADHD]), you will want to contact a professional outside the school setting who specializes in the assessment of learning, academic, behavioral, and cognitive issues.

Depending on what your child may need, any of these professionals might be appropriate. Keep in mind that the first person you contact may not be the one who ultimately provides the treatment. You may find that you eventually have two clinicians involved in your child's care, such as a psychiatrist who prescribes medication and a psychologist who provides treatment, or a psychologist who provides individual therapy to your child and a social worker who provides family therapy. Regardless of the clinician's specialty, finding the right clinician is difficult, and unfortunately, there are no hard-and-fast rules. However, here are some tips to keep in mind when you are in the process of finding a clinician:

- Word of mouth is often the best source of information. Pediatricians, school psychologists and counselors, and teachers are often tuned into the best clinicians in your area. Asking them "Who would you see if your child had a problem?" usually gets a frank and helpful response. Friends can also be a wonderful resource, but be sure to consider the source. What works for one family may not work for another.
- Medical schools and university psychology departments that operate clinics often provide very good care, although you may be seen by a psychiatrist or psychologist in training who is supervised by a senior staff member. In this case, you will want to obtain information about the clinician providing the direct service and the supervisor's experience and quality of supervision.

- Check out the clinician's credentials. A good rule of thumb to keep in mind is the more complex your child's problem, the more training and experience you will want from your clinician.
- Make sure your clinician is licensed in his or her chosen field. You want to make sure that the person you see is licensed in the state in which he or she practices or that the person you see is supervised by a licensed professional (typically in the context of a training program such as a psychiatry residency or a psychology internship).
- Ask about how much experience the clinician has. Again, the more complex the problem, the more important it is to get a more experienced professional.
- Ask about the types of therapies or evaluations the clinician is competent to perform and make sure it is a good match with what your child or family needs.
- Most importantly, trust your instincts! I cannot count the times that parents have come to me for a second opinion, bemoaning the fact that they did not have a good feeling about the first professional they consulted, but they went ahead and saw him anyway. Just because you have gotten a referral from a reputable source, you will not necessarily find that the referred clinician is right for you. Personality counts in this arena, and you need to have someone you connect with—someone you immediately trust and to whom you relate.

There are also a few things not to do when you are searching for a clinician. First, it is rarely ever a good idea to get a name from the phone book or the Internet. Second, it is almost never a good idea to see a therapist who is treating one of your relatives or close friends. An exception to this rule is when you are just seeking a neuropsychological or educational evaluation (such as for a learning disability) or when you are seeing a doctor who is primarily providing medication. Finally, do not get caught up in having a prescribed idea as to what type of demographic qualities the therapist should have, such as a certain gender, age, or religious preference. Although some children do need and benefit from seeing either a male or female therapist, most children will do fine with either one. Same goes for age— many times parents want a young therapist who can relate to their child or an old therapist who can act as a surrogate grandparent— but it is much more important for you and your child to find that personal connection, and personal connections are rarely based on demographic qualities alone.

WHAT TO EXPECT FROM THE EVALUATION PROCESS

Whether the first clinician you see is a psychologist, psychiatrist, social worker, or pediatric neuropsychologist, he or she will first spend time talking to you and to your child. Your clinician will have

---

Where Does My Child's Pediatrician Fit in This Process?

Pediatricians are often the first professional you will consult when your child has a mental health problem. Some pediatricians are quite good at determining what the problem is and helping you figure out what your next step should be (e.g., therapy, medication). Other pediatricians prefer to handle things on their own, sometimes taking a wait-and-see approach or giving you a quick prescription. They may have limited knowledge about the usefulness of therapy and specialized psychological assessments. Some pediatricians (although these are few in number) do not know much about mental health concerns at all and may have a tendency to downplay your concerns or overreact to the situation. It is quite likely that your pediatrician is adept at determining the problem and figuring out the next step, but if he or she is not, you should feel comfortable seeking other opinions.

---

to consider many issues simultaneously to understand your child's problems and make a diagnosis. The issues he or she will be considering include the child's emotional, behavioral, cognitive, and social functioning as well as the environmental factors that contribute to the child's problems. The clinician will also be taking into account how gender, age, and cultural factors influence the child's symptoms and behaviors. The assessment itself can range from a *clinical interview* with the parents and child to more *structured behavioral assessments* or *psychological testing*. Clinical interviews are most common and include talking to the parents about the problem and taking a comprehensive developmental history. Behavioral assessments typically involve observing the behavior as it occurs in the home or school settings. Examples of this might include the school psychologist observing the child during class or on the playground. Psychological testing includes giving children standardized tests that measure their cognitive, academic, or personality functioning. In some cases (in fact many would argue this is the ideal), a multidisciplinary approach is used and involves assessing information from different informants and using different methods, such as interviews, observations, and tests. Furthermore, the assessment process may involve talking with the school or your child's teacher.

Regardless of the ultimate format of the evaluation, a clinical interview is nearly always part of the process. During the interview process, the clinician will meet with you and your child separately and, often, together. The purpose of the interview is to gain basic information about the problem from the perspectives of you and your child (if the child is old enough). Expect the clinician to ask about your child's development, medical history, family history, social relationships, academic history, and your expectations, hopes, and concerns that you have for your child. A good interview will not only focus on weaknesses but also on a child's strengths and positive qualities. Interviews are most often *unstructured,* meaning the clinician will ask questions in a flexible manner, but sometimes a clinician will use a *semistructured* format in which he or she will ask specific questions in a consistent manner. If, during the course of the interview, the clinician perceives that certain areas of functioning deserve greater scrutiny, he or she might suggest a more comprehensive evaluation. For example, if a child is performing poorly in school, the clinician might suggest pursuing testing that would evaluate this issue. Sometimes, in the course of the initial interview, the clinician may conduct a *mental status exam* in which the clinician asks questions of the child and observes the child's appearance, thought processes, mood, cognitive functioning, and awareness of his or her surroundings. Overall, it is important to keep in mind that the purpose of this process is to understand the child's particular problem in a way that can directly the appropriate diagnosis and treatment.

STEPHEN: A BOY WITH MULTIPLE ISSUES

Stephen was a 9-year-old fourth grader who was referred for an evaluation because he had difficulty paying attention in school, symptoms of depression, and problems with reading. He had had poor attention skills since kindergarten, and his family had experienced a number of significant stressors that were thought to contribute to his difficulties, most specifically the death of his mother when he was in second grade, after a long illness that began when Stephen was a preschooler. Because Stephen's household was quite disrupted for much of his life, his teachers thought that his problems with attention and academic skills were due to the traumatic experiences in his home life. However, his fourth grade teacher was concerned that although family stress might be a contributing factor, it might not be the only reason he was not progressing in school.

Stephen's teacher discussed Stephen's difficulties with his dad and suggested they pursue an evaluation with a child psychologist who could possibly shed light on Stephen's difficulties. When Stephen and his dad arrived for their first appointment with me, I spent much of the time talking to Stephen's father. His father reported on Stephen's birth and early life history. Stephen was a happy boy for much of his early life. His developmental milestones, such as walking and talking, were appropriate. Once Stephen reached preschool, though, teachers complained about his difficulty staying seated during circle time and his problems learning letters. Soon after, Stephen's mother was diagnosed with cancer, and his grandmother came to live with them to take care of the family while his mother underwent treatment. Stephen's home life became a mixture of confusion and chaos as his mother's health declined.

During the clinical interview with the dad, I asked about Stephen's school history and discovered that Stephen had difficulty learning to read and was described as "the worst reader in the class." He continued to have problems paying attention, staying seated, and behaving impulsively, both at home and in the classroom. His father noted that Stephen reminded him of himself as a child because he was "always getting into trouble" and "never was a good reader." More recently, Stephen complained of stomach aches when it was time to go to school. He appeared sad and sometimes even angry, and he began to have problems with his peers. Stephen's father also reported that Stephen had difficulty sleeping.

When I spoke to Stephen, I found a boy who had difficulty staying with a particular topic for any length of time. He was frequently out of his chair and was in constant movement. He became particularly agitated when he was asked about school, and it was obvious that this was a difficult topic to discuss. He denied feeling sad or anxious, but he did admit to having trouble sleeping, and he was very reluctant to talk about his mom. At the end of the session, I spoke to Stephen and his dad together. It was obvious that there was much pain about the loss of Stephen's mother. Both Stephen and his dad appeared to be depressed, and although they seemed to desperately want to communicate, neither had the ability to move beyond his pain to a place where they could discuss their losses.

After completing a full assessment, I felt there were three problems that needed further exploration. First, Stephen was exhibiting symptoms consistent with ADHD, and his problems with reading suggested the possibility of a reading disability. I referred Stephen for neuropsychological testing to determine whether an attention deficit or learning disability was the cause of his difficulties in school. Second, I felt that Stephen and his father could benefit from family therapy, and I made a recommendation for family therapy. Third, I thought that the emotional and attention difficulties Stephen was experiencing warranted at least a consultation with a child psychiatrist to determine whether medication could be useful in treating these symptoms. It is fortunate that all of the professionals I referred Stephen to were part of the same hospital setting, and they were able to collaborate on their findings. This is not always the case, but you should expect professionals to collaborate with one another regardless of whether they work in the same setting. Results of the neuropsychological evaluation did indeed indicate the presence of a reading disability and ADHD. As a result of the evaluation, Stephen's father contacted Stephen's school and an individualized educational plan that included tutoring in reading and strategies to help him cope with his attention problems was developed for him. The family therapist helped Stephen and his dad identify and articulate the causes of their sadness. She taught them more effective communication skills, and they became more emotionally expressive and responsive to each other at home. Finally, the consultation with the child psychiatrist indicated that Stephen's difficulties would respond quite well to medication, and medication was pursued.

One year following his initial evaluation, Stephen was reporting no symptoms of depression and few feelings of hopelessness. His reading skills had improved as a result of individualized tutoring, and his attentional problems were significantly helped with medication. He was participating in activities and interacting with his friends. He and his dad had found that although they would always feel the loss of Stephen's mother, the two of them finally felt like a family who could meet the challenges that would come their way.

WHAT ARE THE COSTS OF THESE TREATMENTS?

The cost of treatment varies considerably depending on how complex your child's problem is and where you live. The cost of an initial evaluation with a psychologist or psychiatrist will likely be in the range of $250 to $600, depending on how long the appointment lasts. Hourly rates for psychologists can range between $100 and

What Questions Should I Ask the Professional Who Might Be Evaluating My Child?

Do not be afraid to ask questions of a prospective clinician. Competent professionals will be happy to answer questions you may have about their qualifications, and you should be wary of professionals who do not. Typical questions that I hear include the following:

- How many years have you been a psychologist?
- Where did you get your training?
- What will you do if my child needs further treatment (such as medication)? Is there someone to whom you typically refer?
- What type of assessments do you perform? What types of treatments are you competent and trained to do?
- How many children like my son or daughter have you seen before?
- Do you have a particular area of expertise?
- Are you a solo practice or are you part of a larger network?
- How do you handle emergencies?

$250 per hour (or more if you live in an expensive metropolitan area such as New York City). Other caregivers such as social workers typically charge less. If you are pursuing psychological testing or neuropsychological testing, a full neuropsychological battery can vary widely from $2,000 to $5,000, depending on the complexity of the evaluation and the area of the country in which you live. Educational evaluations typically cost much less, ranging from $800 to $2,000.

Of course, the issue of insurance always arises when considering treatment. There is no hard-and-fast rule for insurance coverage. It really depends on your particular plan, with some plans paying for unlimited therapy sessions (this is rare) and others covering a specific number per year (this can be as few as eight sessions per year). Further complicating this issue is the fact that many professionals do not take all insurance policies, so you may find yourself in the situation of finding the perfect clinician but having to pay out of pocket to see him or her. If it has been recommended that you seek a neuropsychological evaluation as part of the evaluation process, you should know that nearly all insurance plans do not cover assessment of school issues. Some plans cover issues related to attention and emotional issues such as ADHD and anxiety. Most do cover issues related to medical problems such as epilepsy, head trauma, brain tumors, or issues related to birth trauma.

HOW DO I GET MY CHILD TO THE EVALUATION?

So you have made the decision to have your child evaluated, but now you find yourself in the difficult situation of convincing your child that he or she needs to go to the evaluation. Sometimes children go willingly; other times, reluctantly; and once in a while, they just refuse to go at all. First of all, you need to take a look at your own feelings about this process. If it took you weeks or even months to become comfortable with the idea of seeking assessment and treatment, you cannot expect your child to embrace the idea in one conversation with you. However, sometimes children do embrace the idea. They have been struggling; they are aware of their struggles; and they are relieved that you have noticed and are going to do something about it. Other times, children are aware of their difficulties, but this awareness is so painful to them that they do not want attention paid to their problems. In this case, they typically do not think anything can be done to help them and, thus, do not feel talking to someone else will help.

Regardless of where your child falls on this spectrum, you need to approach the topic with true empathy. To do that, you need to understand your own feelings about the process. I have heard many parents say to me, "I really don't want my child to come here to see you—I don't want to put her through an evaluation (or have her in therapy)." These same parents will say, "My child won't want to come here to see you," not realizing that their own feelings are being perceived by the child. Children do not like to see their parents in pain, and they also pick up on their parents' feelings and viewpoints and often incorporate them as their own. One way they may "protect" their parents from the parents' own fears or ambivalence about seeking treatment is to collude with them in not wanting to go. Thus, they join with their parents point of view, which creates the scenario in which the parent comes back to me and says, "See she didn't want to go after all." Therefore, the first rule in getting your child on board with the process is to be on board yourself. If this is a particularly uncomfortable or painful process for you, you may want

> There is no shame in seeking psychological help for your child. If your child had strep throat, you would give him or her antibiotics. In a similar vein, if your child is struggling emotionally, finding the right kind of help is exactly the right thing to do.

to spend some time talking to a professional yourself about why this is so difficult. Did you go through a similar experience as a child? Is it just so hard to see your child struggle? Are you worried about the future? All of these issues can be explored and helped by talking to someone.

Sometimes, the parents are quite eager and ready to bring their child into treatment, but the child is just not willing to go. Other kids are willing to go, but they may have questions and concerns. In either case, here are some guidelines for approaching this topic with your child:

- As indicated earlier, approach the topic with an empathic understanding that this might be hard for your child. At the same time, approach this as a problem-solving endeavor. Validate with your child that you have noticed that she is struggling. Do not make too big of a deal of it, but be honest in your assessment of your concerns. It is OK to tell your child that you are confused, nervous, or worried and that you need to get some guidance on how to help him. Sharing responsibility in addressing the problem will help your child feel he is not alone. Let your child know that you need help and that this is not just about figuring out what is "wrong" with him but also about helping you get a better understanding of what is happening so that you can be a better parent.
- Explain to your child what to expect of the process. Let him know that there will not be "shots" with this type of doctor and to expect that this doctor will be asking questions to figure out how best to help him. Give your child information about your role in the process as well.
- Explain to your child whom she will be seeing. If you have gotten the name of a doctor from a friend or your child's pediatrician, let her know that the referring person has confidence

that the doctor he or she recommended can help. You should feel confident about your choice as well. If you are not, your child will not be either.

- Let your child know that he or she has a say in the process and that you are willing to make changes if the process is not helpful for him or her.
- Make sure your child understands that the process is confidential. Friends will not find out about this unless your child tells them.
- Normalize the process. Many, many children seek treatment and evaluations at some point in their childhood, and you can tell your child that this process is quite common. If you or someone you know has received mental health services, let your child know what the process was like and how it was helpful.
- Create an open environment for discussing your child's feelings and concerns. Saying things such as "Well you're going no matter what!" is not helpful. Instead, hear your child's concerns, let her know the concerns are valid, and give her the opportunity to talk about these concerns with you.
- Many clinicians meet with the parents for an initial consultation. If you have done that and you felt comfortable with the clinician, you can tell your child something positive about your experience with the doctor. This can be quite encouraging to your child.

CONCLUDING THOUGHTS

Depending on your child's particular problem, there is an array of professionals with whom you can consult. Finding the right clinician may take some time, but getting recommendations from people you trust, going to a reputable source such as medical schools or university psychology departments, and checking the clinician's credentials can help point you in the right direction. It is important for you to trust your instincts—if you do not "click" with a particular clinician, you should go elsewhere. There is no "one size fits all" with regard to psychological treatment, and you should feel completely comfortable with the clinician you ultimately choose. Feel free to ask questions and make sure you like the answers before committing to a particular clinician. And finally, there is no shame in seeking treatment; in fact, it might be one of the best calls you ever make.

CHAPTER 3

DIAGNOSIS AND TREATMENT: WHAT ARE THE POSSIBLE TREATMENTS, AND HOW WELL DO THEY WORK?

Treatment approaches for children that are based on sound research and clinical knowledge have grown tremendously over the past 25 years. Most interventions are targeted to a specific problem or area of difficulty, such as anxiety or depression, and in Parts II and III of this book, I discuss each of these areas of difficulty and the most effective treatment approaches in depth. However, the point of this chapter is to begin to orient readers to the array of possibilities by highlighting some of the main approaches used with children and their families while taking stock of what is known about the general effectiveness of treatments for children.

More than 550 different treatment approaches are currently in use to help children. It should be obvious that it would be well beyond the scope of this (or any) book to discuss these in detail, but in this chapter, I expose you to the major approaches. Just to confuse the issue, many psychologists who work with children consider themselves *eclectic*—in other words, they use different approaches for different problems and often combine approaches to treat specific problems. These approaches might be best illustrated by looking at Sally, a 9-year-old girl with an anxiety disorder who was referred for psychological treatment by her school guidance counselor.

SALLY'S STORY

Sally's difficulties began about 2 months ago when she started feeling sick at school. She frequently visited the school nurse because her stomach hurt, and she sometimes complained of headaches and difficulty catching her breath. The school nurse typically called Sally's mother, who picked her up from school. This scenario was becoming quite common, and recently Sally sometimes did not come to school at all. At home, Sally would frequently cry in the morning, complaining of a stomachache and nervousness. When Sally stayed home, she spent most of her time watching TV or with her mom. In fact, she had a long history (since preschool) of wanting her mom around all of the time, and she tended to get upset whenever the two of them were separated. However, this difficulty with separation became even worse since Sally's father was hospitalized for a heart attack 3 months ago. At about this time, she began wanting to be close to her mother constantly, appeared anxious and unhappy, and had difficulty sleeping.

Now that you've read Sally's story, let's explore the most common approaches to treatment and see how they might apply to her. The exhibit at the end of the chapter also gives you an overview of how these theories view a disorder such as anxiety.

PSYCHODYNAMIC TREATMENTS

I begin this exploration with psychodynamic treatments for children because they are often what people think of when they think of therapy. The psychodynamic model has its roots with Sigmund Freud. The model proposes that psychological difficulties are the result of conscious and unconscious conflicts. The idea behind the treatment is that by bringing the unconscious conflicts to light, the symptoms might be relieved. With younger children this awareness can occur through play therapy, whereas with older children (as with adults) the awareness occurs by talking with the therapist, who helps to identify the underlying conflicts, which eventually leads to resolution of these conflicts and more adaptive coping skills.

In Sally's case, the therapist would probably use a combination of play and talk therapy that would allow Sally to gain insight into her problem. This process would probably last several months and possibly longer. The therapist might explore Sally's early relationships with her parents, perhaps focusing on her attachments to her mother and father. Discussion of Sally's dreams and early childhood memories along with nondirected play would be used to determine the underlying problem, which could be an insecure attachment to one of her parents or a fear of her own anger. The theory states that once the underlying problems are resolved, the overt symptoms of anxiety, school refusal, and psychosomatic complaints can be resolved.

Unfortunately, there is not strong evidence that this model works well for most childhood disorders, in part because its concepts can be difficult to define and, thus, to research. However, partly in response to the lack of extensive research on the psychodynamic approach, many other psychological models have emerged. Even though these models are quite different from the psychodynamic approach, many psychologists who are not narrowly psychodynamic in their approach will still use that model to conceptualize certain problems, and they will use some of the aspects of play therapy as a way of getting to know the child and understand her emotional problems in a meaningful way.

BEHAVIORAL TREATMENTS

Although psychodynamic therapists believe that psychological problems will diminish as self-awareness grows, behavior therapists doubt that self-awareness is the key. The focus with this therapy is on

Systematic desensitization teaches the child to associate a pleasant and relaxed state with an anxiety-provoking one. Systematic desensitization is commonly used to treat phobias in that the child will learn to associate the fearful object (e.g., spiders) with a relaxed state.

the behavior itself. For instance, a behavior therapist might argue that you can understand why you are depressed, yet still be depressed. Therefore, instead of attempting to alleviate distressing behaviors by resolving underlying conflicts, the behavior therapist applies evidence-based or well-researched *learning principles* to eliminate the unwanted behavior. Such procedures might include systematic desensitization, positive reinforcement, time out, or modeling positive behavior.

In Sally's case, the therapist might target her problem with going to school by setting up a reinforcement schedule (i.e., rewarding her for going to school) and by instructing her parents as to what to do when she refuses to go to school. If Sally has anxiety about going into the school building, the therapist might ask her to develop a hierarchy of anxiety-provoking situations, ranging from school activities that cause mild anxiety to those that are panic provoking. The therapist would then train Sally to relax by teaching her how to relax each muscle group. Then the therapist would ask her to imagine, with her eyes closed, a mildly anxiety-arousing situation; this might be getting into the car in the morning. If imaging the scene caused Sally anxiety, the therapist would instruct her to switch off the image and go to deep relaxation. The imagined scene is repeatedly paired with relaxation until Sally would feel no anxiety while imagining it. The therapist would then target another one of Sally's behaviors until each of the situations in the hierarchy has been addressed. Behavior therapies have been shown to be quite effective at treating a number of psychological problems, most notably anxiety and phobias.

COGNITIVE THERAPIES

The underlying theme of cognitive therapy is that cognitive, or thinking, processes exert powerful effects on our feelings and our behaviors. In other words, what we think affects how we feel and what we do. Thus, many psychological problems stem from powerful *irrational* beliefs. Cognitively oriented therapists believe that psychological disorders stem from problematic or distorted ways of thinking; they believe that if these ways of thinking can be changed, the problematic behaviors can be alleviated. For example, from the cognitive viewpoint, children become depressed because they develop a cognitive *schema* that includes a negative outlook on the future, lack of confidence in their ability to effect change on their environment, and a tendency to blame themselves for problems they cannot control. Depressed children and adults have been found to attend more to negative cues in the environment than positive ones.

During the course of therapy, the cognitively oriented therapist will help the child recognize the irrationality of her views by identifying such beliefs and then helping the child see that these views are distortions of reality. Other times, the therapist may focus on a child's *attributions*—her beliefs about the causes of her own and others' behaviors. Many times children attribute their failures to internal causes, such as their own lack of ability or effort, even when this is not the case. These same children may attribute successes to external causes, such as lucky breaks, even when the success was due to their own efforts. In therapy, the child is taught to perceive successes as resulting from *internal* causes and failure as resulting (at least sometimes) from *external* causes. Overall, cognitive therapies have been shown to be quite effective in treating many psychological disorders, particularly anxiety and depression.

In Sally's case, she may be convinced that if she leaves the house her father will have another heart attack or that if she goes to school her mother will be unable to cope without her. During

43

the therapy process, the psychologist will help Sally change these unrealistic and irrational fears by examining their reasonableness. For instance, the psychologist will help Sally understand that just because she was at school when her father had his heart attack does not mean that her behavior did—or will—affect what happens to her father's health. Helping Sally to develop more rational and more adaptive ways of thinking should help her behavior to change, and she should be able to cope with her feelings of anxiety and attend school.

COGNITIVE BEHAVIOR TREATMENTS

Very often, cognitive and behavioral treatments are used together in treatment. Cognitive behavior therapists view psychological problems as stemming from *both* faulty thoughts patterns and faulty learning experiences. Thus, the psychologist uses techniques from both of these approaches. In Sally's case, the psychologist might first start by examining Sally's faulty beliefs and irrational thinking and help her to replace them with more adaptive ways of thinking. In addition, the psychologist might teach Sally better coping strategies and help her regulate her behavior while teaching her parents how to better respond to her maladaptive behaviors. Overall, the psychologist will help Sally learn to think more realistically and positively and use better coping strategies that will help her get to school and to stay there once she arrives. Cognitive behavior treatments are used very frequently with children and their parents, and some studies have found that using both approaches together is more effective than using one alone.

FAMILY TREATMENTS

Family therapy models assume that the entire family needs to be treated when there is a family member who has problems that are related to family life. There are many types of family therapy, but all of the approaches tend to view a child's individual problems as stemming from problems in family relationships. The therapy process encourages the constructive expression of feelings and the establishment of rules that the family members agree to follow. During therapy, family members gain insight into their problematic patterns of interaction, and with the support of the psychologist, they learn to change these patterns into healthier ones. Often family therapy occurs after one of the family members (sometimes called the *identified patient*) presents for individual psychotherapy. The therapist will try to improve communication and relationships among family members by helping them learn to provide and accept constructive feedback and gain insight into their patterns, potential pitfalls, and strengths as a family. The atmosphere is a positive one in which no single person in the family is blamed for the family's problems.

Family therapists typically use a *systems approach* whereby the relationships between family members (or *family system*) are explored and maladaptive relationships are identified. For instance, in Sally's case it might be possible that the family is overly child focused, or perhaps Sally and her mother are too closely allied together as a result of fear that Sally's father will have another medical emergency.

At other times the psychologist may explore the emotional boundaries between family members. Boundaries that are too rigid or too diffuse can cause problems; what most families need is a flexible family pattern that can shift boundaries when the circumstances call for it. In Sally's case, the psychologist might identify that there was a rigid boundary between Sally and her mother from an early age and that because of this inflexible boundary Sally was unable to cope with her father's illness. The psychologist will work at achieving a balance between enmeshment and disengagement between Sally and her parents in the hope of establishing a more fluid coping style for the family.

Family therapy has been shown to be about as effective as individual therapy when the child's problem is related to the family system and is much more effective than receiving no treatment at all. Quite often it is used in conjunction with individual treatment in that the family will meet with the family therapist while individual members receive treatment from their own psychologists.

BIOLOGICAL AND MEDICAL TREATMENTS

The medical model views childhood disorders as resulting from biological impairments, and thus, it relies on medication and other biological approaches to treatment. Recent studies of brain development and genetics have indicated that many psychological disorders have roots in biological and genetic factors. This information has resulted in using medication for a wide variety of issues, such as using stimulant medications (e.g., Ritalin, Adderall, Dexedrine) to treat attention-deficit/hyperactivity disorder (ADHD), antidepressants (e.g., Prozac, Zoloft, Celexa) to treat depression, antianxiety medications (e.g., Xanax, Klonopin) to treat severe anxiety, and mood stabilizers (e.g., lithium, Depakote) to treat excessive mood swings and aggressive behavior.

Current medical practices are based on a wide range of research findings that have shown that many classes of drugs are effective in treating psychological disorders. For example, both stimulants and certain antidepressants have been found to be successful in treating ADHD in that they help children inhibit their tendency toward impulsivity and enhance their attentional capacities. But to effectively treat the problem, the psychiatrist or medical doctor has to understand key factors such as a child's environment (family, school stressors, social supports), biological (or genetic) predisposition, and the effect of one of these on the other.

Psychologists recognize the importance of biological factors when treating and evaluating children, even though they are not able to prescribe medications (except in a few states and with additional specialized training). Well-trained child psychologists will know when it is appropriate to make a referral to a child psychiatrist for a medication evaluation, will help parents negotiate this process, and will consult with the psychiatrist about the child's case as needed. Many medications have been shown to be quite effective at treating childhood disorders, and I explore this in more detail in Chapter 15. Although medication is effective in many cases, it is generally more effective when used in conjunction with psychotherapy.

In Sally's case, the psychologist may have made a recommendation to a psychiatrist, who might consider medication to treat her symptoms of anxiety and possible depression. Both psychotherapy (particularly cognitive behavior treatments) and medication have been shown to be effective in treating anxiety problems, and children with anxiety disorders appear to respond to the same medications as adult patients do. Overall, the use of medication to treat children's psychological problems has grown in the past 20 years, and this is resulting in increased awareness and acceptance of these medications as part of a holistic treatment process.

COMBINED TREATMENTS

More often than not, psychologists will use two or more of these interventions to treat children. As mentioned previously, a child like Sally may participate in psychodynamic or cognitive behavior treatment while also receiving medication. Children with ADHD may take stimulant medication while receiving special behavioral therapy techniques within the classroom. A child with depression because of a family stressor may receive medication, individual therapy, and family therapy. As you read through Parts II and III of this book, keep in mind that many children have features of more than one disorder (such as anxiety and depression), and many therapists use more than one treatment approach.

SO HOW EFFECTIVE ARE THESE TREATMENTS?

Efforts to evaluate treatment effectiveness have increased significantly over the past decade, but there is still much work to be done. Overall, the news is good. Children who receive psychotherapy report greater decreases in negative symptoms than children who do not receive therapy. The average child who is treated for a particular disorder is about 75% better off than the average child with the same disorder who does not receive treatment. Treatments tend to be just as effective for children who experience internalizing disorders such as depression and anxiety as they are for children who exhibit externalizing disorders such as ADHD and conduct problems. The treatment effects tend to be long lasting, and generally, the longer the child is in treatment, the more improvement is seen in his or her symptoms.

Overall, there is no doubt that child psychotherapy has a positive impact on the lives of children and families. Study after study has consistently demonstrated that children who receive treatment outperform children who are waiting for treatment and children who receive a placebo treatment. Furthermore, in many studies it is becoming clear that some forms of therapy work better than others. Thus, the world of psychology is at the point now at which one can conclude that therapy works for children, but there is still much to learn about how well specific treatments work for specific disorders. In the next two parts of this book, I help you sort out this question. Even though therapists are still learning and pediatric psychological studies are ongoing, there is still a wealth of information that you can use to determine what to expect when seeking treatment for your child.

Overview of Theories of Anxiety	
Psychodynamic	The focus is on unconscious conflict possibly relating to conflicts in relationships with parents that are unresolved and/or unconscious suppression of feelings such as anger.
Behavioral	Avoiding a feared stimulus becomes a learned response that serves to maintain the child's fear even when he or she is not exposed to the stimulus.
Cognitive	An anxious mind-set distorts threats in the environment, and poor problem-solving ability is exhibited.
Family	Family factors and parenting practices such as overinvolvement, overprotection, and modeling of anxiety contribute to the child's anxiety.
Biological	Certain brain systems are over- or underactive in children with anxiety disorders.

CONCLUDING THOUGHTS

It may feel as if there are an unlimited number of treatments available to children—psychodynamic treatment, cognitive behavior therapy, family therapy, and medical treatments are available to treat many different problems. As I mentioned before, there is not one "perfect" treatment, and most psychologists will employ more than one type of treatment. The effectiveness of each of these treatments varies, but children who receive therapy do better overall than children who do not receive treatment. Regardless of the treatment used, it is important to feel confident in the competence of the psychologist. There are many paths to a healthy outcome, and there are a number of treatments from which to choose so that you can feel comfortable with the one that feels right for you and your child.

Part II

COMMON CHILDHOOD DISORDERS

CHAPTER 4

ATTENTIONAL AND DISRUPTIVE BEHAVIOR DISORDERS

Brandon was a hyperactive first grader who was having trouble mastering basic academic tasks because he could not stay focused long enough to hear what his teacher was saying. Lydia was a 14-year-old freshman in high school who was so disorganized that she was getting Cs and Ds in her classes because she couldn't turn in her homework on time. Adam was a somewhat angry 12-year-old who refused to comply with his parents' requests for him to be home by curfew, and when his parents gave consequences for his misbehaviors he became angry and negative.

All of these very seemingly different problems are referred to as *externalizing* problem behaviors. Externalizing problems, or problems that put children in conflict with others, can include a mix of impulsive, hyperactive, inattentive, aggressive, and delinquent acts, although it is important to note that most children with externalizing problems do not fall on the delinquent end of the spectrum. In fact, the vast majority of them will display symptoms of inattention, hyperactivity, or impulsivity that are indicative of an attention disorder. In this chapter I review the three most commonly observed externalizing problem areas: attention-deficit/hyperactivity disorder (ADHD), oppositional defiant disorder (ODD), and conduct disorder (CD).

WHAT IS ATTENTION-DEFICIT/HYPERACTIVITY DISORDER?

ADHD is one of the most common, and some might argue one of the more impairing, childhood disorders. Approximately 3% to 5% of school-age children meet criteria for ADHD. Many times I have been asked if ADHD is overdiagnosed. Interestingly, research has shown that it is both over- and under-diagnosed. In other words, there are some children who are diagnosed with ADHD who should not have been. They actually may have other disorders such as a learning disability or an emotional disorder that may cause their behaviors to look like ADHD, or they may not have any disorder at all but are given the label of ADHD anyway. At the same time, research shows that particularly girls with attention problems are underdiagnosed because their problems do not generally cause difficulty for anyone but themselves. Lydia, who was described previously, was one such case. Year after year, her teachers referred to her as "spacey," "disorganized," and "inattentive," but she was not evaluated for ADHD because it was thought these behaviors were under her control and because she was not causing problems with her classmates. Obviously, there is still confusion, at least within clinical practice, about this diagnosis! Part of the confusion comes from the fact that ADHD often co-occurs with other disorders (I talk about this later in this chapter) and that there are different subtypes of ADHD.

According to the *Diagnostic and Statistical Manual of Mental Disorders* (4th ed., text rev.; American Psychiatric Association, 2000), there are three types of ADHD:

- ADHD, predominantly hyperactive/impulsive type, describes children who primarily have problems with hyperactivity and impulsivity.
- ADHD, predominantly inattentive type, describes children who primarily have problems paying attention. Sometimes these children will be referred to as having attention-deficit

disorder even though this term does not exist as an actual diagnosis.

- ADHD, combined type, describes children who have a combination of the attention and hyperactive/impulsive symptoms. Most children with ADHD fall in this category.

As you might have guessed from these three subtypes, children with ADHD tend to have problems with impulsivity, hyperactivity, attention, and distractibility. ADHD is much more common in boys than in girls, in fact, somewhere between 3 to 6 times more common, although some researchers have indicated that perhaps girls are underdiagnosed because their symptoms do not typically cause as many problems for others, and therefore girls may not be referred as frequently for evaluation.

Academic performance in children with ADHD is frequently compromised because their problems with attention and organization (another feature of the disorder) tend to interfere with their ability to perform in the classroom because so much of classroom learning depends on a child's ability to attend. Children with ADHD may have difficulty starting an activity; others may jump into an activity with gusto, only to find their attention quickly waning and their enthusiasm gone soon after they start the activity. They often have trouble organizing their ability to do complex tasks such as term papers or projects. Many children with ADHD cannot inhibit their responses to things in the environment. They have trouble filtering out stimuli as simple as a bird flying past the classroom window or their classmate tapping his pencil. Many parents describe their children with ADHD as "hit or miss" in that sometimes they do something perfectly, and other times they rush through a task without even reading the directions. This may have something to do with their interest level because children with ADHD can be quite attentive when they are interested in a topic or activity. In fact, many current researchers view ADHD as a problem with *flexibility* of attention in that children with ADHD only pay attention to things that are intrinsically interesting to them and tend to have difficulty with things that are not.

This may look like a motivational problem to parents, but it is not. Instead, the compelling nature of the task helps stimulate the attentional system in a way that keeps the child aroused and engaged. People without ADHD can work on a boring task when they have to because their attentional system (which includes the frontal lobes of the brain) is working at its capacity, whereas people with ADHD work best on tasks they have chosen and on tasks they find interesting because their attentional system is underaroused. This is why many parents will say to me, "He can't have ADHD because he plays his video games for hours!"

Because children with ADHD have difficulty inhibiting their responses, interrupt others, have problems waiting their turn, talk before they think, and begin a task before listening or reading directions, they have trouble in school. These same behaviors can lead to trouble with peers, and a fair number of children are "rejected" by their peers because they are intrusive, are not aware of social boundaries, are impulsive, and have difficulty playing by the rules both within the classroom and outside of the classroom. Sometimes, this rejection leads to a loss of self-esteem.

The exhibit that follows lists the criteria of ADHD. To have the diagnosis of ADHD, the symptoms must be present before age 7 years. If a child begins exhibiting these symptoms "out of the blue" in adolescence, the symptoms would be attributed to something other than ADHD, such as depression, anxiety, or stress. These symptoms also have to be present in more than one situation, so if a child exhibits these symptoms at home but not at school, the problem may lie in the home environment rather than in the child. Similarly, if a child is struggling with these problems only in school, the issue might

Symptoms of Attention-Deficit/Hyperactvity Disorder

Inattentive symptoms include the following:

- makes careless mistakes and does not pay attention to details;
- cannot sustain attention in school or play activities;
- does not listen when someone is talking to him;
- cannot follow through on instructions and doesn't finish tasks;
- cannot organize tasks or homework assignments;
- avoids, dislikes, or does not engage in tasks that aren't interesting or require sustained effort;
- frequently loses things;
- is easily distracted; and
- is frequently forgetful.

Hyperactive/impulsive symptoms include the following:

- is fidgety,
- cannot stay seated in activities where being seating is expected,
- runs around in situations in which that behavior is inappropriate,
- cannot play quietly,
- is often on the go or "driven by a motor,"
- talks excessively,
- blurts out answers inappropriately,
- cannot wait his turn, and
- frequently interrupts others.

be due to a poor classroom environment, bad teacher match, or a learning disability that is causing the child to "cope" with his problems by acting out or by not paying attention to his schoolwork. These problem areas have to be impairing—in other words they have to interfere with the child's functioning in at least two different environments (such as home and school)—and six or more symptoms of either inattention or hyperactivity need to be present.

HOW IS ATTENTION-DEFICIT/HYPERACTIVITY DISORDER ASSESSED?

A diagnosis of ADHD should be made after a careful assessment of the child's history and after getting data from multiple informants, such as parents and teachers, across multiple settings, such as school and home. A 20-minute discussion with a psychiatrist is not typically adequate for making a diagnosis of ADHD. Instead, the evaluation should at a minimum include a thorough history and parent and teacher rating scales. Ideally the evaluator will also include tests that measure attention, organization, and other executive function skills. If medication is going to be prescribed, the evaluation should also include a medical evaluation. Because ADHD can look like other disorders (kids with anxiety or depression can also have problems with attention), it is important to rule out other possibilities for these behaviors. Finally, 20% to 30% of children with ADHD also have learning disabilities, so if ADHD is present, it is often a good idea to evaluate for learning disabilities as well.

Executive Functions

Executive functions are the processes in the brain that are responsible for guiding, directing, and managing cognitive, emotional, and behavioral functions, particularly during active novel problem solving. They represent an umbrella construct that includes a collection of interrelated functions that are responsible for purposeful goal-directed problem-solving behavior. You might think of these processes as the organizational part of the brain that allows individuals to be self-aware, plan, monitor their behavior, evaluate their behavior, remember what it is they are supposed to be doing, and be flexible in their thinking and behavior.

WHAT ARE THE BEST TREATMENTS FOR ATTENTION-DEFICIT/HYPERACTIVITY DISORDER?

There are a variety of treatments that have been well validated to treat ADHD. The best treatments include medication, behavior therapy, parent training, and school interventions. Not all of these treatments are used by every child, but they represent the range of possibilities that have been shown to be effective.

Medication

There are a number of scientifically sound and tested treatments for children with ADHD, but many parents struggle with the most well researched treatment modality of all— medication. Literally hundreds of studies have been conducted on children, and the overall results indicate that medication, when properly and carefully prescribed, is the most effective treatment for managing symptoms of ADHD. Stimulant medications are the most commonly used medications to treat the symptoms of ADHD, but several other medications are also sometimes used, such as certain antidepressants and antihypertensives. A lengthy discussion of the pros and cons of these medications is beyond the scope of this book, and the reader is encouraged to consult the reading list in the Additional Resources section at the end of this book for more information about psychiatric medications in children.

There are three classes of stimulants approved by the Food and Drug Administration for use in children with ADHD: the amphetamines (such as Adderall and Dexedrine), the methylphenidates (such as Ritalin, Focalin, Concerta, and Metadate), and magnesium pemoline (Cylert). One other popularly prescribed drug called Strattera is a nonstimulant medication that was developed to treat ADHD. Of the drugs mentioned, Ritalin is by far the most commonly prescribed. Medication has been found to be significantly helpful to about 80% of the children with ADHD in that they have improved attention, are more persistent at tasks (particularly those that are not intrinsically motivating), show less motor activity and restlessness, are more attentive to academics within the classroom, are less impulsive, and are more productive. Medication can also have a positive impact on children's social behavior and on their relationship with their parents because there tends to be less conflict. However, stimulants do not address all of the problems that children with ADHD have. It will not necessarily make children more organized or help them plan their term paper in advance. In addition, some children show little response to the medication (or cannot tolerate the side effects, which can include sleeping problems, anxiety, and poor appetite), and some parents do not want to use medication. Fortunately, there are other important interventions, such as behavior therapy, parent training, and school-based interventions. In fact, some psychologists and researchers have argued that these other interventions should be implemented before trying medication, and they should of course remain in place as needed once the child is on medication. This is an issue to explore with your doctor because each child and family has different needs. The important thing to keep in mind is that there are a variety of options from which to choose and that the choice of options may vary over time depending on the child's needs.

Behavior Therapy

Behavior therapy treatments have been shown to treat symptoms of ADHD effectively when implemented in the home, classroom, or even summer camp settings. In each of these settings, the parent or teacher and child set realistic goals, determine a reward system, carefully monitor the child's performance, and reward the child for meeting his or her goals. Poor behavior may be punished through losing privileges or having a time-out. Psychologists are frequently involved in establishing behavior therapy approaches in both home and school settings.

Parent Training

Parent training applies behavioral approaches to family functioning. It targets not just the child's behaviors but also parenting skills such as teaching parents how to use effective language and to establish appropriate rules in the home, how to use punishment effectively (such as time-outs and other appropriate consequences), and how to reward positive behavior effectively.

School Interventions

Many studies have demonstrated the benefits of behavioral procedures within the classroom environment. These interventions can take the form of academic interventions (e.g., tutoring in specific subjects or teaching organizational or study skills) or classroom interventions such as the posting of classroom schedules and rules, point systems for positive behaviors, or daily report cards (teachers send home a daily note about the child's behavior, which parents can then reinforce at home). Research has also indicated that peer tutoring and computer-assisted instruction can increase attentiveness and decrease disruptiveness.

Combination Treatments

A couple of very important studies have indicated that for some groups of children a combination of behavior therapy with medication is more effective than medication alone. In addition, lower doses of medication are required to achieve the same results when it is combined with behavior therapy compared with medication alone. Throughout it all, the importance of good parenting skills should not be underestimated because parents have an important role to play in their children's development.

Who Can Provide These Types of Treatments?

Medication can only be provided by a medical doctor or nurse practitioner, although in a few states psychologists can prescribe medication under a doctor's supervision. Check http://www.apa.org for more information concerning what is applicable in your particular state.

Behavior therapy is typically provided by psychologists or other mental health specialists.

Parent training is typically provided by psychologists, family therapists, or other mental health specialists.

School interventions are typically provided by school psychologists and school guidance counselors.

Supportive Treatments

Supportive treatments include interventions such as family therapy, individual supportive therapy for the child, and ADHD support groups. Although there is limited evidence that these treatments eliminate or decrease the symptoms of ADHD, they can be useful in helping parents cope with their child's symptoms. Becoming involved in a *support group* can help parents feel they are not alone and provides a forum for them to obtain information from others such as appropriate referrals to qualified professionals, how to help teachers and school administrators understand their child, how to handle the embarrassment of having a child who may be disruptive, and the general stress and frustrations that can be involved in parenting a child with ADHD. *Individual counseling* for the child can help him cope with the inevitable stress and self-defeating patterns of behaviors that can come with ADHD. It can help children identify their strengths and learn adaptive ways of coping with their symptoms. *Family therapy* can help the entire family cope with the blame and anger that can occur when a child has ADHD. Siblings may feel neglected because their parents are "always" managing the child with ADHD, and the child with ADHD may feel overly focused on and criticized, which can set up a negative family dynamic. This type of therapy can help all of the family members develop new skills and attitudes as well as a shared vision for their family's future.

WHAT ARE OPPOSITIONAL DEFIANT DISORDER AND CONDUCT DISORDER?

The first time I met Michael's mother, she came into my office in tears. "You won't like my son," she said.

> He is in the car in the parking lot and refusing to come in to see you but this is nothing new. Yesterday he wouldn't get dressed so I took him to kindergarten naked thinking that once we pulled up to the school he'd hurry up and get dressed. But that didn't faze him at all. He just sat there and refused to get out of the car.

When I asked her about a "typical" day for Michael, she replied,

> A typical day is one where he gets up on the wrong side of bed. He doesn't like the cereal we have and won't get ready for school. He annoys his sister all day long and blames her when he gets in trouble. He can argue with me about anything—his socks are too "itchy" or he doesn't want to wear a coat even when it is freezing outside.

Michael's mother was clearly at her wit's end and was coming for assistance to see how she could help Michael get control of his behavior.

Mark, age 13, was referred to my office for an evaluation because he had just set his third fire, and this time the fire led to several thousands dollars worth of damaged furniture. He had been suspended from school for breaking windows and spray painting graffiti on the outside of the school building. When confronted with what he had done, he lied and denied any wrongdoing. One of his teachers suspected that he had stolen money from her purse. Mark's parents were wondering if a military school was the answer because their local public school was unwilling to take him back unless he got help.

Michael and Mark both show signs of *conduct problems* or *antisocial behaviors*. Children with conduct problems display a wide variety of rule-breaking and disruptive behaviors. The behaviors can range from swearing and temper tantrums to stealing, truancy, vandalism, and assault. These types of behaviors are those that violate family and societal expectations and the rights of others. The nature, causes, and outcomes of children with conduct problems can be quite variable, ranging from minor disobedience to criminal activities. These behaviors tend to be more common in boys than girls during childhood, though the gap narrows in adolescence.

Conduct problems are considered an externalizing behavior problem and consist of two related dimensions of behavior—delinquent behaviors and aggressive behaviors. Delinquent behaviors are those that involve breaking the rules—either family, school, or societal rules. They can include behaviors such as running away from home, setting fires, stealing, using illegal drugs, and committing vandalism. Aggressive behaviors include those behaviors that show aggression toward others, such as fighting, defiance, threatening others, cruelty, bullying, and assault.

WHAT IS OPPOSITIONAL DEFIANT DISORDER?

Children with ODD display patterns of behaviors that include negativity, hostility, and defiance that are above and beyond what is expected for a child of that age. Children with ODD frequently argue with adults, lose their temper, are often angry and resentful, do not comply with adult rules, annoy others, and blame others for their problems. These behaviors are almost always present at home and sometimes at school and in other settings. ODD is more common in boys than in girls before puberty but equally common after puberty. Symptoms are typically present by age 8 years. It is important to remember that these symptoms need to be severe enough to interfere with a child's day-to-day functioning to receive a diagnosis of ODD. Most adolescents display these behaviors at one time or another, but they would not meet the criteria for this disorder.

Parents have to deal with these problems much more frequently than teachers. Typically these children reserve their worst behaviors for those they know well. It can be a difficult disorder to diagnose because these children do not always show signs of the disorder in the psychologist's office. When asked why they act the way they do, they often blame their parents, teachers or other adults for their issues. It is common to hear adolescents with ODD say things such as "If my parents weren't so strict, I wouldn't be acting this way." Sometimes these children can be so convincing that the psychologist or teacher believes that the parent really is the problem! This is rarely the case, however.

ODD typically begins before age 8 and rarely begins later than early adolescence. Quite often parents will report a long-standing history of temper tantrums, moodiness, and low frustration tolerance. As youngsters, these children are often described as having a "difficult temperament," and it is true that some children with difficult temperaments do grow up to have ODD—particularly if they are a poor match for their family environment. In other words, a child who might have been described as "spirited" and who was born into a quiet, placid family might not fit in with the family's dynamics, and thus, the parents might have difficulty understanding their child or making the necessary adjustments (within the family system) to that child's temperament. Often ADHD is present, but not always. Sometimes children with preexisting depression or mood disorders can display these behaviors, and if that is the case, the mood disorder is considered the primary diagnosis. Often, when the depression is treated, the oppositional behaviors go away. Overall, children with ODD tend to have higher rates of comorbid disorders, social impairments, and family dysfunction.

HOW IS OPPOSITIONAL DEFIANT DISORDER ASSESSED?

When a diagnosis of ODD is suspected, the psychologist will initially want to conduct a thorough assessment looking at the child's developmental history (including developmental milestones, medical history, family history) and school history (including how the child's behaviors impacts him or her in the classroom setting). It is important for the psychologist to clearly assess the situations and environmental triggers that can be contributing to the child's oppositional behaviors. Do these behaviors only occur at home, at school, or during unsupervised play times? Are there certain people in the child's environment with whom he is more likely to exhibit these behaviors? For instance, are the behaviors worse with dad, mom, teachers, coaches, or peers? Are there any types of situations that can trigger these behaviors?

Because there are many factors that can contribute to a child's acting-out behaviors, it is not usual for the psychologist to request further testing, such as psychological testing or neuropsychological testing. This testing can be useful in determining the child's cognitive and emotional strengths and weaknesses; the development (or lack thereof) of executive functions skills such as planning, organization, and flexibility; language skills; social skills; and problem-solving skills. For example, Michael, who was described at the beginning of the chapter, was referred for a full neuropsychological evaluation.

The results of the evaluation indicated that he had a nonverbal learning disability, which may make him prone to difficulties interpreting nonverbal cues in the environment and transitioning from one activity to another. He also displayed difficulties with working memory skills in that he had difficulty remembering what he was supposed to be doing. When Michael's mother asked him to go up to his room, get his white socks and blue sneakers, and bring them downstairs, it was too much information for him to remember. He wasn't necessarily being defiant when he came down from his room without his socks—he really could not remember all of the information he was asked to remember. Through this evaluation his parents gained a better understanding of the factors that contributed to his oppositional behavior, and his therapist could use this information to guide her treatment.

Most children with ODD do not meet criteria for nonverbal learning disability; however, most of them do a display a particular cognitive style that makes them prone to oppositional behaviors. For example, researchers such as Dr. Kenneth Dodge at Duke University have found that aggressive children tend to have deficient information-processing skills in regard to social situations; they misperceive social situations in particular ways. For example, they misinterpret or underuse social cues in the environment. They misattribute hostile intent to their peers. On problem-solving tasks, they tend to generate fewer solutions to problems. Surprisingly, they expect to be rewarded (not punished) for aggressive behaviors. This style makes them prone to making bad decisions (because they have misinterpreted what has gone on in the environment) or not making the right decisions (because they have not generated enough ways to solve the problem). Acting aggressively might have been the only solution they thought of, and at the same time, they might think their solution "solved" the problem and expect to be rewarded for their efforts.

Children With Oppositional Defiant Disorder

Children with ODD exhibit the following behaviors:

- have extreme difficulty complying with the limits set by others,
- are frequently argumentative and angry,
- have difficulty controlling their temper,
- display angry and vindictive behaviors,
- have negative behaviors that are usually directed at someone else (most often an authority figure), and
- do not display behaviors that are indicative of major antisocial violations.

HOW IS OPPOSITIONAL DEFIANT DISORDER TREATED?

Many different types of treatment have been used to address children's ODD behaviors. Some programs have focused on changing the discipline techniques of the parents that have contributed to the development of oppositional behavior and poor parent–child interactions. These programs teach skills such as use of time-outs, use of appropriate language, and how to use reinforcement and consequences. Other programs have focused on the cognitive factors underlying the child's behaviors. Dr. Ross Greene at Harvard Medical School incorporated a number of intervention strategies into a cognitive behavioral model of intervention called collaborative problem solving. This approach helps the parents understand the parent and child characteristics that contributed to the development of the oppositional behaviors, makes parents aware of the strategies for handling unmet needs or expectations (e.g., parents can impose their *will* by forcing the child to do what they want him to do, collaboratively problem solve with the child, or remove the expectation that the child behave in a different way; some of these strategies work better than others), helps parents understand how each one of these strategies impacts parent–child interactions, and helps parents learn how to use collaborative problem solving as a way to resolve disagreements and oppositionality. Recent research over the past decade has shown this model to be quite effective.

It is important to keep in mind that children with ODD can vary considerably, and there is no one-size-fits-all approach. A child whose problems are fueled by poor language comprehension is going to need a different approach from one whose problems are fueled by a coexisting depression. Thus, it is important to work with a psychologist who has expertise in working with these children so the psychologist can individualize the treatment on the basis of your child's particular needs at that particular time.

WHAT IS CONDUCT DISORDER?

CD is a more severe form of ODD. Children with CD go even further in violating the basic rights of others. They are aggressive to the point of being cruel to persons or animals; they destroy other people's property; they lie, cheat, skip school, defy their parents' rules, and run away from home. Stealing, shoplifting, forgery, breaking into homes or businesses, and harming others can all be part of this diagnosis. This disorder usually begins by age 10 years, and this is referred to as *childhood-onset type*. In some cases the child shows no problems until after age 10 years, and this is referred to as *adolescent-onset type*. Children with a milder form of this disorder often improve over time, but in severe cases these symptoms can persist into adulthood. It is more common in boys than in girls. Children with CD often have other comorbid (or coexisting) disorders such as depression, anxiety, substance-related disorders, learning disabilities, and ADHD. It is important to note that most children with these other disorders do not develop CD but that many children with CD do develop or already have another disorder as well.

Although no one knows definitively what causes CD, genetic and biological factors as well as households with significant family conflict have been identified as possible causes. CD is more common in households where there are parents with alcohol or substance dependence or mood disorders; this does not mean that every child with CD grows up in this type of home. Some researchers have also observed that the high rates of family conflict in children with CD may be the result of parenting a child with behavior problems, rather than the cause. For example, Mark, who was mentioned at the beginning of this chapter, grew up in a home where it was "dad's way or the highway." Sometimes dad's way included physical punishment such as spanking with a paddle or a belt. In fact, Mark's father told me, "If my wife had let me hit him more, we wouldn't be in this situation." Unfortunately, physical punishment has not been found to be an effective treatment strategy for children with CD, and in fact, Mark's father might have made things worse.

HOW IS CONDUCT DISORDER ASSESSED?

As is the case when assessing ODD (described previously), the psychologist will need to use multiple assessment methods to assess CD. These can include interviewing the parents, child, and teachers; having parents, child, and teachers complete behavior ratings scales; and directly observing the child or adolescent in the home or school setting. Even though the child has the "problem," the psychologist will spend more time interviewing the parents than the child. This is because children (especially children under the age of 9 years and children with this disorder) are not very good at reliably reporting their symptoms. In other words, children with conduct problems do not usually think they have a problem. However, the psychologist will definitely take time to talk directly to the child to get the child's understanding of why he has been brought to treatment and to get his perceptions of his parents' concerns and what his family life is like.

When the conduct problems involve classroom performance, interviewing the child's teacher or teachers is essential, and if this is the case, the psychologist will ask for written permission to communicate with the teacher. The psychologist will also typically ask whether the child is taking any medication and get a developmental history to determine whether a medical or temperamental issue

> Major symptoms of CD include the following:
>
> • aggression toward people and/or animals,
> • destruction of property,
> • deceitfulness or theft, and
> • serious violation of rules.

might be contributing to the behaviors. The psychologist will also want to rule out the possibility that the child has a coexisting condition such as depression, anxiety, or ADHD. Many children with CD have problems with peer interactions, and this is an area that should also be assessed. Finally, if the conduct problems appear to be connected to school performance, it is important that a more thorough evaluation of the child's academic, intellectual, and neuropsychological functioning be pursued. I have many times conducted neuropsychological evaluations of adolescents with a diagnosis of CD, only to find out that they had suffered from an undiagnosed dyslexia or learning disability. The roots of their oppositional behavior could be traced to the fact that school was unusually difficult for them, not because they were not trying hard enough but because they could not read or write. Thus, when assessing externalizing behaviors, a comprehensive approach to the assessment is imperative.

HOW IS CONDUCT DISORDER TREATED?

Generally, the earlier a child receives treatment (particularly before 13 years of age), the better the outcome. *Family interventions* are one of the more effective treatments for CD. In these types of interventions, parents are taught more effective ways of managing their child's behavior. In addition, parents and children typically meet together in this model so that the psychologist can teach them better and healthier ways of expressing feelings and interacting together. *Community-based residential* programs for adolescents have also been found to be effective when the problems are more severe. In this model, the adolescent lives in a group home while attending his or her local school. The treatment includes behavioral procedures (such as rewards and punishment), social skills training, academic tutoring, and home-based services. The treatment may also include family therapy to help facilitate the adolescent's transition back home. *Skills training* assumes that children with CD have a deficit in one or more basic skills that can include behavioral, cognitive, or emotional problems. The child is then taught these skills within the therapeutic setting. Finally, medication can be useful in treating a co-occurring problem such as ADHD or depression. Research on children with CD indicates that most children with the disorder will have it (or at least aggressive behaviors) for a long time, and so intensive treatment that incorporates a combination of behavioral and family approaches is important.

CONCLUDING THOUGHTS

It is probably clear from reading this chapter that children with externalizing problems can vary widely from common and highly treatable mild problems to more severe, but much rarer, problems that could include criminal behavior. Most children with externalizing issues don't fall at the more severe end of the spectrum. Similarly, it is probably clear that there are many forms of treatment, ranging from medication to parent guidance to various types of therapy. What is most important is that the treatment is tailored toward a child's and family's individual needs and developmental level and that these often change as the child matures and moves through different developmental stages. The treatment approach that works well for a 4-year-old does not apply to a 14-year-old. Finally, if you suspect your child has ODD or CD, be sure to ask your doctor to look for other problems such as depression, anxiety, ADHD, post-traumatic stress disorder, learning disabilities, or an undiagnosed medical condition because it is important to get treatment for these co-occurring conditions as well.

CHAPTER 5

AUTISM AND PERVASIVE DEVELOPMENTAL DISORDERS

The disorders discussed in this chapter differ in some ways but are similar in one important way: Each is characterized by problems in a number of areas of development, particularly social interactions, communication, and/or stereotyped behaviors. The most common of these disorders are autistic disorder, Asperger's syndrome (AS), and pervasive developmental disorder (PDD). These disorders are typically apparent early in a child's development (within the first few years of life). Often these disorders are referred to as *autism spectrum disorders* because they are thought to exist along a continuum, with the defining feature being a pervasive difficulty in the ability to relate to others. These disorders can range from the more severe form of autism to the much milder diagnosis of AS.

WHAT IS AUTISM?

Children with autism have significant problems with social interactions and communication and a very restricted repertoire of activities and interests. The problems with social interactions are very severe (not just being shy or a bit aloof) and include (a) difficulties with nonverbal behaviors, such as very poor or nonexistent eye contact; (b) an inability to recognize others' feelings (or even recognize the presence of another person); and (c) problems establishing or maintaining friendships (to the point of being unaware of others' needs or presence). Children with autism also have problems with communication that can include delayed speech, unusual speech, or problems comprehending the speech of others. *Stereotyped behaviors* or repetitive behaviors are observed in children with autism, and these behaviors can include rocking, a fascination with objects that spin, a fascination with a simple object such as a string, or a preoccupation with parts of objects (e.g., a button, a specific part of the body). To meet criteria for a diagnosis of autism, a child must have a significant delay or abnormal functioning in one of these areas before the age of 3: social interaction, language (particularly language used in social communication), or imaginative play. Most children with autism have never had a period of normal development, although some parents do report normal development until the age of 1 or 2 years.

In addition to the diagnostic criteria for autism that are indicated in the following example, there are a number of other associated problems that many (but not all) children with autism exhibit. Although it is not necessary to have these difficulties to receive a diagnosis of autism, many children with the disorder have difficulties in the following areas:

- an unusual oversensitivity or undersensitivity to simulation such as light, noise, touch, or smells;
- intellectual ability—although children with autism show a wide range of intellectual skills, about 75% will show problems in intellectual functioning; and
- adaptive behavior—children with autism tend to show problems coping with day-to-day living skills, or *adaptive* functioning, which include skills such as dressing, personal grooming, and the ability to get along well with others.

Features of Autism

Impairment in social interaction that can include problems with

- nonverbal behaviors (e.g., poor contact),
- developing normal peer relationships (e.g., problems making and keeping friends), and
- the ability to reciprocate socially or emotionally with others (e.g., an inability to share in the excitement or happiness of others).

Difficulties in communication that can include

- a delay in language or a lack of communication skills (such as not speaking in sentences until age 4 years or not using any words until age 2½ years),
- problems sustaining conversation (e.g., not being able to make small talk or even sustain any type of a conversation with peers),
- repetitive or unusual language (e.g., mixing up pronoun use, referring to oneself in the third person), and
- play skills that are nonexistent or inappropriate for age (e.g., trouble with imaginative play).

Unusual patterns of behavior that can include an

- abnormal preoccupation with certain objects or a restricted interest in certain objects (e.g., things that spin),
- an adherence to usual rules or routines (e.g., a need to line up all of their toys in a particular order),
- repetitive motor movements (e.g., hand or arm flapping, finger flicking)
- an overwhelming preoccupation with parts of objects (e.g., being interested in how the door of a toy car opens rather than using the toy car as a whole play object).

HOW IS AUTISM ASSESSED?

Early identification of children with autism is key because the sooner a child is evaluated, the sooner early intervention can begin, and early intervention is key to the best possible outcome. Because autism is a diagnosis that can affect many areas of functioning, a comprehensive assessment is typically warranted. A comprehensive evaluation can include interviews with the child's parents and caretakers; direct observation of the child in the doctor's office and at home or school; and tests of intelligence, language, and day-to-day living skills. The evaluator may ask you to complete forms that measure symptoms of autism, and he or she may complete a structured observation of your child. The Autism Diagnostic Observation Schedule uses activities to assess whether the child displays behaviors relevant to autism, for example, by engaging the child in telling a story or in playing a game and seeing whether she is able to be engaged or even able to do these activities.

WHAT ARE THE EFFECTIVE TREATMENTS FOR AUTISM?

Children with autism have been shown to benefit considerably from early, intensive, comprehensive programs. Comprehensive programs for children below the age of 5 years typically include behavior therapy such as applied behavior analysis, speech and language therapy, occupational therapy, and social skills training. Research has shown that children can make significant gains in these types of programs and that these gains are typically maintained years later. Programs shown to be successful for children of any age with autism have a number of common elements: a focus on communication, attention, and social skills; a highly structured school environment with a low student-to-teacher ratio; a predictable home, school, and therapy environment; and a high level of structured family involvement. When parents are more involved in the treatment process, children are more likely to generalize and maintain what they learn in school and in therapy. The most effective treatments are ones that are very intensive in that they are given for many hours per day and in different environments (e.g., at home and at school). Some children may need behavior therapy to address concerns such as self-stimulation, aggression, and tantrums. Social skill facilitation has also been found to be effective, particularly if this facilitation occurs through the school day in addition to in structured therapy groups.

Unfortunately, there are no magic bullets or pills that can treat autism, although medication can be useful in treating some of the associated symptoms, such as inattention, aggression, and self-injurious behavior. Some children with autism may have seizure disorders, and medication is used to treat these conditions. Finally, research has shown that many types of treatments are not very helpful in treating the underlying causes of autism. These include vitamins, auditory and visual training exercises, skills patterning, and functional communication.

Are Rates of Autism Increasing?

The idea of an "autistic epidemic" has been expressed in both the psychological literature and in the media. Rates of autism have increased; this is in a large part due to better detection. Research has also documented that as rates of autism have risen, rates of mental retardation (also known as *intellectual deficiency*) have decreased; in other words, psychologists and other mental health diagnosticians are more likely to diagnosis autism, perhaps in part as a result of the increasing social acceptance of a diagnosis of autism or PDD as compared with a diagnosis of mental retardation. One controversial issue is that rates of autism are increasing because of mercury in children's vaccines. To date, research has clearly demonstrated that there is no connection between vaccination and autism. In fact, rates of autism have actually increased in countries that discontinued the use of mercury in vaccines.

WHAT IS ASPERGER'S SYNDROME?

The incidence of AS is thought to be about 1 out of every 500 children in the United States, and it occurs more often in boys than in girls (about a 4:1 ratio). AS is considered to be part of the autism spectrum, and some children who are eventually diagnosed with AS had more classic symptoms of autism as toddlers or preschoolers, but many of their symptoms were remediated with intensive services to the point that they no longer meet the full criteria for autism. However, most children with AS never appear as seemingly autistic but instead display behaviors such as poor eye contact, difficulty interacting with others socially, restricted patterns of behavior (e.g., an intense preoccupation with specific subjects), and problems understanding pragmatic language (e.g., difficulty understanding slang expressions or realizing when someone is teasing them). The example of Jill, a 7-year-old with AS, illustrates these points.

Jill was described by her parents as being a "difficult child from Day 1!" Her early history was significant for problems with fine and gross motor skills, frequent temper tantrums, problems separating from her parents, and difficulty going to sleep at night. In preschool, Jill was described as a "loner" who "never shared or played with other children," although her language and cognitive skills appeared to be above average for her age. In kindergarten she was noted to be an anxious child who had "sensory issues" in that she "didn't like the sounds of the gym" and would cry when things became noisy during gym class. In first grade, the school psychologist suggested that she participate in a social skills group where she could practice learning how to communicate and get along better with others.

Jill's parents came in for an evaluation because they were concerned that Jill was unable to cope with the demands of elementary school. Despite participating in the social skills group, Jill continued to struggle with social relationships. She invaded people's personal space by getting too close to them; she was unaware when people were trying to avoid her or tell her to stop; and she obsessively focused on her own interests. These interests included an intense preoccupation with Beanie Babies and Webkinz. They were nearly her only subjects of conversation, and in addition, she had a flat, odd way of speaking and a difficulty understanding the perspectives of others. A comprehensive evaluation indicated that she met criteria for AS, and her parents were actually relieved to know that there were many resources available to them to help Jill.

Children with AS have problems in two major areas: social skills and patterns of behavior (meaning their patterns of behaviors are restricted to particular interests to the point of being odd or obsessive). Their problems in these areas cause them to have significant impairment in social or school functioning. In terms of social skills, to get the diagnosis, problems need to occur in at least two of the following areas of functioning:

- problems with nonverbal behaviors, such as poor eye contact or an inability to use or understand appropriate facial expressions;
- problems developing age-appropriate peer relationships;
- problems in the ability to share their interests or achievements with others; and
- a lack of the ability to give and receive social and emotional information.

In terms of behavior patterns, children with AS exhibit at least one of the following behaviors:

- a preoccupation with an interest that is abnormally intense (often these interests are quite unusual for a child's age, e.g., being interested at age 5 years in ancient Roman coins or being obsessed with a particular cartoon show at age 10 years);

- inflexible adherence to routines or rituals;
- repetitive motor movements (e.g., hand flapping); and
- an preoccupation with parts of objects.

In addition to these issues, many children with AS also have difficulties in some of the areas described in the paragraphs that follow.

Cognitive skills: Children with AS can have problems with some aspects of problem-solving skills because they can have trouble "seeing the forest for the trees" or pulling information together from multiple sources. They can have trouble learning cause and effect and have difficulty getting the gist of movies or books because they tend to be concrete thinkers.

Learning and academic skills: Children with AS can struggle with certain types of learning, particularly with math and reading comprehension because of the difficulty they can have with drawing conclusions or seeing the "big picture." Writing skills can be impaired because some children with AS have difficulty with fine motor coordination and the planning and organizational skills needed to be a good writer. Homework completion can be difficult because of the multitasking needed to complete some homework assignments, particularly project-type assignments. It's not always the case, however, that children with AS struggle with academics, as children with AS can be gifted within the math or writing domains.

Language and communication skills: Children with AS are sometimes gifted within the verbal realm. They can talk about their particular topics of interest as if they are college professors or "little adults," which of course isn't appealing to their peers. Despite strong verbal skills in some areas, children with AS can have difficulty understanding figurative speech or jokes. The may have difficulty with social communication skills (also known as *pragmatic language skills*), and they may speak in an overly formalized, detailed style (also known as *pedantic speech*). For example, Garth, was a fourth grader who used vocabulary that many adults had difficulty understanding! He would correct his teacher's grammar and vocabulary use, and when his peers would make fun of this tendency, he would cry because he couldn't understand why they were "picking on" him when he was "only trying to be helpful to the teacher!"

Social skills: Given that problems in social skills are one of the major criteria of AS, it's not surprising that children with AS can stand out from their peers in a negative way. However, children with AS tend to want to have social relationships with their peers, they just don't know how to go about doing it. They are often delightful with adults and younger children but have difficulty knowing how to make friends with their peers.

Motor skills: Children with AS can have difficulty with fine and gross motor skills, and many children with AS first come to clinical attention through an occupational therapy evaluation for motor skill development. Problems with fine motor skills can lead to problems with handwriting and drawing. However, many children with AS are quite good at drawing. The subject of their artwork, though, can take on a perseverative quality. For example, I have seen many children with AS who would only draw one type of anime character or one type of animal, such as horses.

Sensory issues: Children with AS can reportedly have difficulty with an oversensitivity to sensory stimuli, such as sounds, touch, smells, and taste. For example, children with AS may have difficulty sitting through a movie in a theater because the sound is too loud. They may dislike certain smells, such as the school lunchroom, to the point that they feel (and sometimes) get sick. They may be unable to wear all but the most "broken in" or softest clothing.

HOW IS ASPERGER'S SYNDROME ASSESSED?

AS can be diagnosed through a clinical interview, but because of the associated symptoms reported previously, it is thought best for a child to have a more comprehensive evaluation such as a neuropsychological evaluation that includes measures of intellectual functioning; educational ability; visual–motor skills; language skills (particularly pragmatic language); executive functions; and social, emotional and behavioral skills. Reports and rating scales from parents and teachers should be included as part of the evaluation, and it is often helpful for the evaluator to complete a classroom observation of the child.

WHAT ARE THE BEST TREATMENTS FOR ASPERGER'S SYNDROME?

Social skills training is typically recommended for children with AS because of their well-documented social difficulties. Individual psychotherapy (particularly cognitive behavior therapy) can be useful in treating problems with social reasoning, anxiety, or obsessive tendencies. In addition, children with AS often benefit from additional therapies as appropriate:

- occupational therapy for children who have difficulty with fine motor skills,
- physical therapy for children who have difficulty with gross motor skills, and
- speech and language therapy for children who have difficulty with pragmatic language.

Within the classroom environment, children with AS benefit from a structured, organized environment with a low student-to-teacher ratio. A small percentage of children with AS need the more comprehensive services of a full-time classroom aide. Some children need direct tutorial instruction in specific academic areas such as math, reading comprehension, written expression, or executive function skills. Medication can also be warranted to treat cooccurring symptoms of anxiety or inattention.

WHAT IS PERVASIVE DEVELOPMENTAL DISORDER NOT OTHERWISE SPECIFIED?

This may seem confusing, but the previously discussed disorders— autism and AS—are considered types of PDD. What can be even more confusing to parents is that sometimes clinicians will diagnose children with autism/PDD. Parents may find themselves asking, "Which is it?" In theory, the actual diagnosis of PDD not otherwise specified is used when there is a severe impairment in the development of social or communication skills or when a child has stereotyped behaviors, but the criteria for autism are not fully met. The diagnosis is also used for cases of *atypical autism*—children who do not meet full criteria because of their age of onset or because their symptoms are not quite severe enough. Although they have autistic-like behaviors, they either have too few symptoms or the wrong pattern of symptoms.

Similar to children with autism, children with PDD have problems with social skills. They have difficulty connecting with others and may have delayed speech. They typically have reduced eye contact and problems reading social and facial cues. They may also engage in repetitive or stereotyped behaviors.

HOW IS PERVASIVE DEVELOPMENT DISORDER ASSESSED?

PDD is assessed in much the same way that autism and AS are assessed. However, it can be difficult for a psychologist to differentiate between these disorders, and this is because aspects of these disorders overlap with one another. Because a high number of children with PDD have cognitive impairments, it is important for the child to receive a comprehensive evaluation—preferably a neuropsychological evaluation along with consultation with a pediatric neurologist—that includes tests of cognitive, academic, language, and neuropsychological functioning.

HOW IS PERVASIVE DEVELOPMENT DISORDER TREATED?

Because PDD is so similar to autism, the treatments are also similar. Behavior therapies, social skills training, and school interventions are the most commonly used strategies. Medication can be helpful, and although there is no standard treatment regimen, medication is used to treat cooccurring symptoms such as anxiety and inattention.

CONCLUDING THOUGHTS

One of the most confusing things for parents with children who have symptoms on the autism spectrum is whether they have, or even can get, an accurate diagnosis for their child. It is common for two different evaluators to come to a different decision. One may say your child has "high functioning autism," whereas another may say your child has "Asperger's." Sometimes the diagnosis is given because it is the best label that can be used to advocate for your child. The important thing to keep in mind is that the treatments for all of these conditions are similar because they are all considered autism spectrum disorders. These behaviors fall on a continuum, and your child's symptoms may fall at different places on the continuum depending on the setting and your child's age.

CHAPTER 6

MOOD DISORDERS

Maurice, a 12-year-old boy, came into my office because he told his parents "Sometimes I just feel like hurting myself . . . I want to jump out of the window or suffocate myself with my pillow." Over the past few months, Maurice had become more and more withdrawn and sad. Although he used to have friends, now he was described by his teacher as "a loner who never smiles and seems very troubled." Maurice had difficulty maintaining what used to be "stellar" grades because he had difficulty concentrating and felt unmotivated. At home, Maurice was having trouble sleeping, ate compulsively, and complained of stomachaches and other minor physical complaints, such as headaches. He had difficulty getting along with his parents and seemed irritable most of the time.

Tara, age 16 years, was brought to the hospital emergency room because she had threatened her father and was acting "bizarre." Tara's father indicated that she was moody "all of the time"; whereas sometimes she was sad and sullen, at other times she was full of life and extremely energetic. When she felt "full of energy," Tara needed little sleep and never felt tired. At these times, she talked incessantly, appeared hyperactive, and felt "out of control." Periodically, Tara thinks about hurting herself, although this was the first time she had thought about hurting someone else. She arrived at the emergency room frightened by her thoughts, and she and her family were confused as to what to do.

Maurice and Tara exhibit fairly severe cases of what are called *mood disorders*. Most children with mood disorders do not display the severity of symptoms that Maurice and Tara do, but most do seem constantly unhappy, show little enthusiasm for many things, are moody, or think "life is just not worth living." For example, Benny was a 12-year-old who had never felt suicidal but who was chronically sad and who did not often feel up to hanging out with his friends. His sad mood made it difficult for him to complete his homework because he sometimes just felt too tired and lethargic to get things done. Benny was diagnosed with and treated for a mild depression. Mood disorders are one of the most common psychological disabilities in children, affecting about 6% of children at any particular time.

Mood disorders fall into two broad categories. At one end of the spectrum are the children who experience *depression*. These children typically experience prolonged (more than 2 weeks at a time) bouts of sadness. They frequently have lost interest in activities and friends. However, some children, particularly teens, do not appear outwardly sad. Instead, they express their depressive symptoms through their irritable mood, and they may seem grouchy, cranky, touchy, or easily upset. In fact, irritability is one of the most common features of depression and is present in almost 80% of children with depression.

The other category of mood disorders includes children who experience *mania,* during which they may be grandiose, talkative, hyperactive, and display poor judgment. They may even seem *euphoric* in that they have an exaggerated sense of well-being. Children who display an ongoing combination of extreme highs and extreme lows may have a condition known as *bipolar disorder* (which used to be referred to as *manic-depressive disorder)*. Children who have bipolar disorder may have alternating periods of feeling high and low, or they may feel both extremes concurrently.

WHAT IS DEPRESSION?

Depression refers to feelings of unhappiness that are far more severe than the occasional blues or the normal mood swings common to all people. All children diagnosed with depression or a major depressive disorder experience either a depressed mood or a loss of interest or pleasure for at least a 2-week period. In addition, they also experience at least five of the following symptoms:

- significant weight loss or weight gain or decrease or increase in appetite nearly every day,
- insomnia or hypersomnia (too much sleep) nearly every day,
- overly active or agitated (i.e., very restless) or not active enough (i.e., can't get off the couch to do anything) nearly every day,
- fatigue or loss of energy almost every day,
- feelings of worthlessness or guilt (i.e., Why did I do that?) almost every day,
- problems concentrating or a tendency toward indecisiveness almost every day, and
- thoughts of death or suicide (with or without a specific plan).

It's not unusual for depression to be overlooked in children because people tend to view childhood as a happy time, and it can be difficult for caregivers to think that children can be depressed, even when they are exhibiting depressive symptoms. Surprisingly enough, depression can even occur in preschool children, and it can take the form of physical symptoms and complaints (e.g., my tummy hurts, I don't feel well) or sometimes acting out in an aggressive way. As children age, hopelessness can be an indication of depression. For example, Maurice, who was described at the beginning of the chapter, felt that it didn't matter what he did because he would still feel like a failure. His parents would point out his strong intelligence and his talents, but he would reply, "It doesn't mean anything because we're all just going to die anyway." Another indicator of depression in children is a sudden and unexplained drop in academic performance or social participation. Although many children who experience school difficulties are not depressed, when school or social difficulties come on rather suddenly—without a history of problems in school or with friends—depression may be a possible explanation.

Depression affects about 2% to 5% of school-age children and adolescents, and generally, the older the child, the greater the risk of depression. Until adolescence, depression is equally common in boys as it is in girls, but by about age 13 years, it is more common in girls, who represent about 65% of cases. Depression does tend to run in families; children who have a parent with depression have up to 3 times as great a risk of becoming depressed themselves.

My Child's Doctor Said My Child Has Dysthymia. What Is That and How Is It Similar to Depression?

Dysthymia is diagnosed when children display depressed mood for most of the day, for most days for at least a year. They tend to be irritable or unhappy most of the time, and although their symptoms are chronic, they are less severe than those seen in children with major depressive disorder. It can be difficult to distinguish dysthymia from major depressive disorder, particularly in children, and some experts have raised the issue of whether it is a true mood disorder or a personality characteristic. In fact, it is sometimes referred to as the "Eeyore" disorder after the sad donkey in *Winnie the Pooh*. Dysthymia is a risk factor for later major depressive disorder. In other words, children with dysthymia often go on to develop more serious depressive symptoms, so it is important to get the right treatment for dysthymia, which can include therapy (particularly cognitive behavior therapy), medication, or a combination of the two.

HOW IS DEPRESSION ASSESSED?

Special tests do not need to be used when evaluating a diagnosis of depression. Instead, the doctor (frequently a psychologist or psychiatrist) will spend time talking with you and your child. The psychologist may ask you to complete rating forms that ask questions about your child's behavior in different domains. These types of rating forms ask whether your child has experienced changes in her sleeping or eating habits, and you may be asked to rate these changes on a scale from 1 (*no change*) to 5 (*severe change*). The psychologist may also ask your child to complete self-report forms such as the Children's Depression Inventory. These questionnaires provide the clinician with information about which symptoms are most prominent and what beliefs the child holds that seem to be contributing to her symptoms. Sometimes, the psychologist will suggest *projective testing,* which includes measures such as the Rorschach (sometimes known as the *Inkblot Test*) or the Children's Apperception Test. These types of tests are used when there is an unanswered question regarding the child's behavior or feelings about a situation. Common questions include "Is my 8-year-old depressed because I just divorced his father?" "Is my teenager still struggling with the death of his mother 4 years ago?" "Why is my child depressed when everything seems so good in his life?" The reasons for suggesting projective testing can vary widely, but the goal is generally to focus on why a child is depressed.

During the process of assessing whether a child is depressed, the psychologist may ask the child questions that sometimes make parents uncomfortable. These kinds of questions include "Have you ever felt so bad that you thought life was not worth living?" "Have you ever wished you were dead?" If children answer yes to questions such as these, the psychologist may continue the line of questioning by asking, "Have you actually thought of hurting yourself?" "What did you consider doing?" If a child has reached the stage of forming a suicide plan, it is important for the psychologist to determine what the plan is, how likely it is that the plan would be implemented, and how dangerous the possibility. For example, I evaluated Kenny, a depressed 6-year-old, who said that he had a plan to kill himself by poking himself "with a really pointy pencil." Although I was concerned about his level of depression, I wasn't concerned that he would actually be successful in hurting himself. Brianna, another depressed 6-year-old, responded to my questioning by telling me that she fantasized about running into the freeway near her house. Needless to say, I felt Brianna was in need of more intensive services. I was similarly worried about Jared, a 16-year-old boy who told me that "when he killed" himself it would "be in the car in the garage with the motor running." When assessing these symptoms, it was important for me to determine how recent these thoughts were, under what circumstances they occurred, and how persistent and severe they were. Jared's symptoms were severe, but they tended to occur only when he faced a lot of stress. Thus, monitoring his stress level was very important.

Parents frequently are uncomfortable with professionals asking questions about suicide. In fact, they are often afraid that asking the question might cause their child to be suicidal. This issue has been studied, and there is no indication that talking about these issues causes suicidal ideation. Furthermore, in severe cases, assessing suicidal ideation helps professionals protect children at risk of self-harm. Most children are frightened by their suicidal feelings and will feel relief that someone had the courage to ask about them. Asking children about what stopped them from carrying out their plans can help professionals determine the elements of hope and ambivalence about death that can be used therapeutically. For example, some children say they could not commit suicide because it is against their religion, whereas others feel distress at what it would do to the people they love. These reasons can be used as coping mechanisms—

using the child's religious beliefs as a way to cope with symptoms of depression or focusing on the love a child has for his parents—within therapy.

WHAT ARE EFFECTIVE TREATMENTS FOR DEPRESSION?

Psychotherapy is most often the first treatment that is used when treating children with depression. Although more traditional, insight-oriented therapies can be helpful, research has shown that more active, cognitive-based approaches are most effective. These approaches are explained in more detail in Chapter 12. These approaches work on changing the child's perceptions and belief systems. However, sometimes children refuse to participate in therapy, and sometimes therapy does not work as quickly as one would like it to. Other times, the depression is so severe that there is concern that the child might hurt herself. In those cases, medication can be quite useful. These options are discussed further in Chapter 15, with the most commonly prescribed drugs for depression in children being Zoloft, Paxil, Prozac, Luvox, and Celexa. When children exhibit depression along with another disorder, the psychiatrist may want to try a drug that treats both disorders. For example, for children who have attention-deficit/hyperactivity disorder (ADHD) and depression, Wellbutrin may be the drug of choice. It is important to work with a competent professional, typically a child psychiatrist, when medication is used to treat depression in children and adolescents.

Overall, various therapeutic approaches (medication and psychotherapy) have been found to be very successful in treating depression in children and adolescents. The most important thing is to seek treatment. The more serious the depression, the more active the approach should be. For example, if your child has a more mild depression, you might want to start by seeking psychotherapy treatment. However, if your child's depression is moderate to severe, pursuing both psychotherapy and medication might be the best course of action. Similarly, if your child's depression is not responding to psychotherapy after a period of 2 or 3 months, you should consider a medication consultation. Even if your therapist does not raise the issue, do not be afraid to ask your child's therapist if she would benefit from medication in addition to therapy. Depression typically feels hopeless for the person experiencing it and can lead to hopelessness in other family members as well, but treatment does work.

Suicide

The risk of suicide exists when a child has a mood disorder, and the risk tends to increase as the child gets older. Most children and adolescents with depression report suicidal thinking, although only 16% to 30% of children who think about killing themselves actually attempt it. Drug overdose and wrist cutting are the most common methods, but they are (fortunately) not the most effective methods. Those tend to be the use of firearms, hanging, or suffocation followed by poisoning or overdose. Although girls attempt suicide more than boys, because they do not tend to use guns, they usually do not complete the suicide. One of the biggest risk factors for completed suicide is access to guns, and under no circumstances should a depressed child (particularly an adolescent boy) have access to firearms. The risk of suicide tends to be greater when

- the child has been getting more and more depressed over a period of time;
- the child has less communication with others, particularly when communication with others has recently broken down and there is a major loss, such as a breakup with a boy- or girlfriend or best friend; and
- there is a history of self-injurious behavior, such as cutting.

WHAT IS BIPOLAR DISORDER?

In the past, bipolar disorder was not thought to occur in children. Research conducted over the past 10 to 15 years has indicated that it does indeed occur in children, but it can look quite different than adult-onset bipolar disorder. In general, children with bipolar disorder show severe cycling mood swings and outbursts. Cycling mood swings occur when a child is up one minute and down the next. During a manic episode a child may display symptoms such as intense irritability or rage, or he may show extremely silly, giddy, over-excited, talkative behavior coupled with grandiose beliefs—beliefs such as thinking he will get an A on a test even though he didn't attend class or study for the test. He may tend to be restless, agitated, and have difficulty sleeping. Sometimes the initial symptoms of bipolar disorder are depression, anxiety, severe irritability, and mood swings. In adolescents, the first symptoms that parents may notice are alcohol or drug use, legal problems (e.g., for shoplifting or assault), or severe relationship difficulties.

Tara, who was mentioned at the beginning of this chapter, displayed many of these symptoms. She had a history of having intense periods of energy when she could focus on one activity for hours at a time. However, she also had periods of time when she was extremely distractible and constantly jumped from one activity to another. In spite of these difficulties, much of the time she said she felt "terrific." Her erratic mood swings did not bother her a bit, and she found her tendency toward reckless behavior to be "exciting." When she was depressed, her depression was typically very impairing, and she was often self-destructive in that she had a history of cutting or scratching herself.

The diagnosis of childhood-onset bipolar disorder is a difficult one to make because children with bipolar disorder can look quite different from adults with the disorder. Professionals may be hesitant to give this diagnosis unless everything else has been ruled out.

Cutting

Recent research has suggested that at least 10% of high school students have experimented with cutting, using razors, knives, fingernails, or other sharp objects to cut their skin. Cutting is a maladaptive coping mechanism for some teens who are experiencing psychological pain. Without more positive ways of managing their problems, they resort to cutting to establish a sense of control and make themselves feel better. These children and teens frequently have depression, anxiety, low self-esteem, or a mood disorder. They may also be impulsive or obsessive, which can make it hard for them to stop cutting once they have started. If you find your child has engaged in this behavior, be sure to share this information with his or her therapist.

Sexual Behaviors Seen in Children With Bipolar Disorder

Although many children with a diagnosis of bipolar disorder do not exhibit sexualized behavior, many do. Preschool and school-age children can show an increased interest in sexual matters that is inappropriate for their age. They may expose themselves to other children, play "doctor" in a way that is abnormal for their age, or have a tendency toward frequent masturbation, especially in public. Adolescents may show an obsessive interest in pornography and increased sexual activity (with a tendency toward reckless, unsafe sex).

In terms of the differences between adult- and childhood-onset bipolar disorder, children commonly are *rapid cyclers*. Adults tend to have long cycles of depression and mania—at least 2 weeks at a time. These long cycles are quite uncommon in children, particularly in children under the age of 8 years; in fact, children can cycle within the same hour. The most common mood change for children is irritability along with prolonged and aggressive temper outbursts. In between these outbursts, the children are often described as chronically irritable or angry. Although many adults with bipolar disorder experience euphoria as part of their manic symptoms, many children do not.

HOW IS BIPOLAR DISORDER ASSESSED?

Many of the assessment techniques described previously in the section on depression can be applied to assessing bipolar disorder, with a clinical interview being the most important component. However, the assessment of bipolar disorders is less well developed. It is important to consult an experienced professional—specifically a child psychiatrist or a child psychologist—if the possibility of a bipolar diagnosis exists because this can be a difficult disorder to diagnose. It sometimes can take a while to arrive at the diagnosis because bipolar disorder may initially present as depression or a very difficult temperament. It is also common for children with bipolar disorder to present with cooccurring problems, such as ADHD, school truancy, academic failure, or substance abuse, and it is important that the evaluator rule out any other issues. It is very common for parents to be asked to complete rating forms, such as the Childhood Mania Scale, that ask parents to rate the possibility of manic and depressive symptoms on a scale from 1 to 5.

Although special tests are not required to make a diagnosis, neuropsychological testing can be useful in ruling out some of the cooccurring disorders, such as ADHD. Such testing can also be used to determine the child's pattern of cognitive strengths and weaknesses and whether the child's cognitive style exacerbates his bipolar symptoms. For example, does the child have trouble integrating visual information to the point that he "misses the big picture?" If that's the case, the child may have difficulty understanding complex information in the real world to the point that he becomes frustrated and loses control. Other children can have a slow processing style that can make it difficult for them to process information quickly. If so, a fast-paced environment might be overwhelming. Still other children with bipolar disorder may have difficulty with executive function skills—skills that include planning, organization, or the ability to shift easily from one task to another. If these issues can be identified, it can helpful in determining the approach to take with particular children.

WHAT ARE THE TREATMENTS FOR BIPOLAR DISORDER?

The most common treatment for bipolar disorder is medication; the most commonly prescribed medications are mood stabilizers (e.g., lithium) or atypical antipsychotics (e.g., Risperdal, Invega, Zyprexa, Geodon, Abilify, Seroquel). Dr. Tim Wilens, a child psychiatrist at Massachusetts General Hospital, has noted that clinicians tend to use the atypical antipsychotics as first-line agents for the treatment of children and adolescents who have bipolar disorder because the drugs not only control the manic symptoms (e.g., explosiveness) but also the depressive symptoms of the disorder. For some children, these drugs can work quickly, within a couple of weeks; for other children, the drug's full effect may not be apparent for 3 months.

Even though medication is the most common treatment, a multi-modal approach that includes medication, therapy, and monitoring of associated problems such as alcohol use or ADHD is necessary. Living with a child with bipolar disorder can be very tough on a family, and family therapy can be helpful. It is also important for parents to become educated about the disorder, and programs that are designed for children and their families that include both educational and psychotherapeutic components are being developed. Many of these treatment programs include the types of cognitive behavioral strategies described in the treatment for depression. Unfortunately, treatment of bipolar disorder in children and adolescents is an under-studied area.

When Tara arrived at the emergency room with her father, she had not been previously diagnosed with bipolar disorder. However, the doctor immediately set her up with a comprehensive evaluation the next week, and after a careful review of her history, her doctor diagnosed her with bipolar disorder and prescribed Risperdal. Tara also became involved in cognitive behavior therapy that focused on learning new coping skills, developing a more positive self-image, and teaching her family ways to lessen turmoil. Within the year, Tara became a much happier and more productive young woman. Her grades were good; she enjoyed hanging out with her friends again; and she joined the tennis team. Her family was functioning in more healthy, effective ways. Even though she did experience periods of sadness, they were brief. As she said to me, "This stuff doesn't take over my whole life anymore because I don't get wacked-out about every little thing."

CONCLUDING THOUGHTS

Mood disorders fall into two broad categories ranging from depression to mania. Depression is the more common of the two and is quite common, affecting 2% to 5% of school-age children and adolescents. Psychotherapy, particularly active cognitive-based approaches, is quite effective, and medication can be used in conjunction with therapy if needed. Bipolar disorder is less commonly observed than depression and can be difficult to diagnose. The most important thing to remember is to seek treatment. Mood disorders are treatable, and no situation is hopeless; so, it is important to find the help you and your child need.

CHAPTER 7

ANXIETY DISORDERS

Anxiety is a basic human emotion. It might not surprise you to know that most children experience a large number of worries, fears, and anxieties over the course of their development. One of the biggest challenges for psychologists when considering a diagnosis of an anxiety disorder is to determine whether a child's fear is normal. Certain fears tend to be more common at particular ages: Fear of strangers is common from 6 to 9 months; fear of scary monsters, at around 2 years; fear of the dark, in 4-year-olds; and social fears, in adolescents. Across all ages, children and adolescents tend to worry about their own and their families' well-being.

Most of the time, age-appropriate fears, such as being afraid of the dark at age 4 years, do not require the attention of a psychologist, unless the fears are intense or continue longer than expected. However, if the fear starts to interfere with a child's functioning, for example, if the child can't go to sleep at night or can't attend school, intervention might be necessary. Each anxiety disorder has different symptoms, but all the symptoms tend to cluster around excessive, irrational fear and dread. To meet the criteria for an anxiety disorder, the anxiety must last at least 6 months so it is not just the relatively brief type of anxiety that is caused by a stressful event (e.g., transferring to a new school). It is also important to note that when anxiety disorders are left untreated, they tend to become chronic conditions. Defining and diagnosing anxiety disorders in children, however, can be complicated, and most children who have one type of anxiety disorder will meet criteria for at least one other type of anxiety disorder at some time. For example, at age 3 years, Jacob couldn't attend preschool because he couldn't leave his mother's side. His problems separating from his mother were so bad that she couldn't leave him for a moment without his having a meltdown. After 6 months of this, she consulted a psychologist, who diagnosed Jacob with separation anxiety disorder (SAD). Jacob received treatment for this to the point that he could attend kindergarten with relatively few difficulties, but during his kindergarten year he began to display symptoms of obsessive–compulsive disorder (OCD). He also presented as generally anxious much of the time, consistent with a diagnosis of generalized anxiety disorder (GAD). Jacob's difficulties aren't as rare as you might think; about 6% to 15% of children will meet criteria for one or more anxiety disorders at one point or another. Children with anxiety disorders also tend to experience other types of impairments, such as poor school performance, social difficulties, depression, and family dysfunction.

In this chapter, I focus on the most common anxiety disorders observed in children. There is a lot of overlap between the disorders, and typically children meet criteria for more than one anxiety disorder. The disorders include

- SAD,
- GAD,
- specific phobia,
- social phobia,
- OCD, and
- posttraumatic stress disorder (PTSD).

It can be difficult to determine which of these disorders is primary, in part because young children often do not know that they are anxious; they may just feel "bad" or be clingy, hyperactive, irritable, or sad. I frequently see children who have been labeled *oppositional* who are actually anxious, particularly when their oppositionality only occurs in new situations or after they have spent an enormous amount of energy holding their anxiety in check. For example, Joachim was a quiet, shy child within his first grade classroom setting. Although he was anxious, he could keep his anxiety under control, at least until he got off the school bus. At that point he would cry, want things "just so," and refuse to eat supper. Joachim was working so hard during the school day not to let his anxiety show that when he arrived home he was unable to control his symptoms.

WHAT IS SEPARATION ANXIETY DISORDER?

You may already have guessed from the title that SAD has to do with the anxiety a child feels when separated from parents or caregivers. It occurs in its worst form when a child reaches school age, but it can be a source of difficulties with babysitters or day-care providers at younger ages. Sometimes, but not always, a precipitating event triggers these symptoms. These events can include a trauma, an illness or operation (particularly if the child is separated from her parents), a move to a new house, or the loss of a pet or loved one. Adam, a 7-year-old whom I treated, lost his grandfather at age 6 when he was in kindergarten. At first, he just complained about going to school because he "missed Papa." Then he started resisting walking to the bus stop, and his mom began driving him to school and walking him into the classroom. Once they arrived at school Adam would whimper and cling to his mother. After much prodding from his mother, teacher, and even sometimes the school psychologist, he would manage to make it into the classroom but then would frequently ask to go to the nurse's office because of headaches or stomachaches; he would explain to the nurse that he felt so sick that he needed to go home. These behaviors were interfering with his ability to function at school. Even when he was in the classroom, he was often worried about his parents' safety, thinking things might be going wrong at home. Adam did, however, respond quite well to cognitive behavior treatment, and by the middle of first grade, he was getting on the bus without any difficulty.

Adam's behavior is typical for many children with SAD. There are certain ages at which children are most susceptible to SAD: kindergarten, the beginning of junior high (around 11 years), and puberty (13 to 14 years). Younger children with SAD tend to be excessive in their need for parental attention. They may cling to their parents during the day and want to sleep in their parents' bed at night. Older children with SAD tend to fear new situations, and they may feign illness or throw a tantrum when their parent leaves. Some children may also become quite dramatic, threatening suicide or acts of self-harm, although it is relatively rare for children with SAD to act on these impulses. Understandably, parents of children with SAD can feel highly distressed by these symptoms.

To receive a diagnosis of SAD, a child must display three or more of the following behaviors; these behaviors have to cause excessive anxiety and be developmentally inappropriate for the child's age:

- excessive anguish when the child is separated from his home or caregiver or when a separation is anticipated,
- persistent worry that a calamity might befall a parent or caregiver (e.g., a parent might become ill or lose his job) or that the parent might die,
- chronic worry that a calamity might lead to a separation from a caregiver,

- reluctance or refusal to go to school,
- fear or reluctance to be alone at home or in other situations,
- difficulty falling asleep without being near a parent or caregiver and/or difficulty sleeping away from home,
- repeated nightmares about separation from parents or caregivers, and
- frequent complaints of physical symptoms when separated from caregivers or when separation is anticipated.

SAD is the most common anxiety disorder in childhood and is found in about 10% of all children. Most children who have SAD have another anxiety disorder—most frequently GAD. Some children (about a third) will also develop depression, and school refusal is common in older children with SAD.

School Refusal

School Refusal occurs when a child refuses to attend school or has difficulty remaining at school for an entire day. It often occurs after a period when the child has spent more time than usual at home with his parent (e.g., illness, vacation) or after a stressful event such as a family move, an accident, or the death of a loved one. For many children, school refusal is really "just" separation anxiety in that the child does not want to leave the parent, although school refusal can occur for other reasons. Most children with school refusal do not have a learning disability or problems with academics that would cause them to dislike school. They may have fears of being bullied by peers, criticized by teachers, or failing, but often these fears have little basis in reality (though, of course, such events should be thoroughly ruled out). Treatment is extremely important because the long-term consequences, such as academic or social problems, can be severe. Treatment usually emphasizes an immediate return to school using cognitive–behavioral techniques, sometimes in combination with medication (antianxiety or antidepressant medications).

WHAT IS GENERALIZED ANXIETY DISORDER?

Louisa, age 12, worries constantly about her schoolwork. She refuses to participate in most of the activities at her middle school because she is worried about what will happen when she is there. After going to one middle school dance, she came home and cried for an hour in the corner of her room because she was worried that no one liked her and that she didn't fit in—despite having fit in quite well. Louisa had chronic headaches, which were extensively evaluated by a pediatric neurologist, but no problems were found. At night, she spent hours making sure her homework was done perfectly. She was an A+ student, but she was never satisfied with her performance and obsessed over every test and every assignment. She had friends, but her anxiety and perfectionism would sometimes drive her friends away. At school, she was a frequent visitor to the nurse's office, complaining of headaches, stomachaches, and minor aches and pains.

Louisa's presentation is typical of a child who has GAD. Children with GAD tend to be thought of as "worry warts." They are constantly worrying about something. To receive the diagnosis of GAD, a child has to display the following symptoms. First, they typically worry about a lot of things most of the time. Children with GAD worry about everything—their family's health, whether the bus is going to be on time, how well they performed on a test, world hunger, the homeless person they passed on the way home from school, the possibility of getting cancer, whether their friends like them, the possibility of earthquakes or tornadoes—the list can go on and on. I once worked with a child who was afraid to go to sleep because she was afraid she might stop breathing and would not wake up. She was also afraid to ride the bus to school because there were no seat belts, and she was afraid of what would happen if she got into an accident. Second, they experience physical symptoms along with their anxiety. Children with GAD feel physical symptoms that can include a pounding heart, restlessness, trouble concentrating, irritability, sweaty palms, stomachaches, headaches, and trouble sleeping. Usually they are bothered by more than one symptom at a time, and the symptoms tend to change according to the situation.

Many adults (at least 5% of the general population) experience GAD, and the symptoms usually begin in childhood or adolescence. If GAD goes untreated until adulthood, it frequently presents with other problems, such as depression or substance abuse. In other words, feeling anxious much of the time (without getting better) can lead to feelings of depression or a tendency to overindulge in alcohol, food, or illegal drugs. Thus, it is very important to seek treatment early, and the available treatments are excellent. GAD tends to run in families, and sometimes there is shame around the diagnosis that is passed down the generations. For example, Mrs. Levin spent much of her life in a state of panic, and when William, her 8-year-old son, started to talk incessantly about his school grades, the fact that his father was traveling frequently for his work (and "could get killed in a plane crash"), and his mother's health (among other things), she initially wanted to downplay his symptoms. As the worries became debilitating (to the point that William did not want to stay at school), she realized he needed treatment but was reluctant to take him because she felt it was "all [her] fault." For much of her life, Mrs. Levin had suffered in an anxious silence, and her symptoms were undertreated. Through the process of bringing William to treatment, Mrs. Levin also received treatment for her own anxiety. This scenario is more frequent than one might expect because it is often the case that in the process of evaluating or treating a child's symptoms, the parents also seek clarification and treatment for their own problems.

WHAT ARE SPECIFIC PHOBIAS?

A *phobia* is an intense, irrational fear of something that is out of proportion for the situation. Many people have minor phobias of things such as spiders, bees, bridges, or elevators, but usually they do not let that stop them from going outside or traveling on a bridge. To be diagnosed with a *specific phobia,* the irrational fear affects a child's quality of life, and the fear of the object or situation becomes so intense that it leads to avoiding particular situations or to extreme anxiety if the situation cannot be avoided. For example, Matthew was intensely apprehensive about getting shots and would throw a huge tantrum whenever it was necessary for him to receive one, so much so that he needed to be restrained by the entire nursing staff at his last checkup. When he was diagnosed with juvenile diabetes, this somewhat minor problem became a life-or-death issue because he needed constant blood monitoring and daily shots. Kevin, a 7-year-old boy, had a fear of dogs that went far beyond what was reasonable; he even refused to visit many of his friends because most of them owned dogs. Unfortunately, his fear of dogs began to interfere with his ability to engage in appropriate developmental experiences, such as playing at a friend's house. For Kevin, avoiding dogs led to a tendency to avoid engaging in friendships—this is where what might have originally been a simple fear crossed the line to become a phobia.

To receive a diagnosis of a specific phobia, children must display the following symptoms:

- The child experiences an irrational, persistent, excessive fear that is cued by an object or situation. For Matthew it was the doctor's office, whereas for Kevin it was the possibility of seeing a dog. For other children it can be an airplane ride, heights, or seeing blood.
- When the child sees the object or is placed in the feared situation, he or she immediately experiences an anxiety response or *panic attack.* In children, the *anxiety response* can include things such as a tantrum, crying, crawling into a ball, running away, or clinging behaviors.

- In adults with panic attack, they recognize that the fear is excessive or unreasonable—in fact this is a criterion for the diagnosis. Children, however, do not always know that their fears are unreasonable; they may think their fears are quite reasonable, and thus, they do not always display this criterion.
- The child will do almost anything to avoid the situation or will endure the situation with intense anxiety.

What is a panic attack? A panic attack is an episode of intense fear or apathy with a sudden onset. The symptoms include feeling faint, nauseous, unable to catch one's breath, and dizziness. The person may feel he or she is "going crazy" or having a heart attack. Often there is no apparent trigger for the attack.

The phobic behaviors mentioned in this list significantly interfere with the child's functioning, development, or relationships.

Psychologists do not know what causes phobias, although some particular theories have been suggested. One theory holds that children with phobias have been conditioned to become fearful of a certain situation or stimuli. For example, a child who was chased or bitten by a dog may then become fearful of dogs in general. Other theories state that children can become afraid of something by seeing someone else display the behavior. I once worked with a child who developed a fear of vomiting in public after seeing someone vomit in a crowd at Disney World. Similarly, a child might become fearful of dogs after seeing someone get bitten by a dog. Other theories state that fears can be learned when adults instruct children to be afraid of certain things. For instance, adults may tell children to be afraid of spiders, bees, snakes, thunderstorms, and more. A parent may say, "Stay away from the bees or you'll get bitten," which (if said frequently enough) may cause a child to have an intense fear of bees.

Phobias are more common than one might expect; about 11% of the population will develop a phobia sometime during their lifetime. Phobias are more common in girls than in boys, and the impact of the phobia on a person's life generally depends on what the phobia is. It's easy to avoid going to the dentist if you're afraid of the dentist, but if you're fearful of dogs or insects, you might find yourself avoiding many different situations, possibly on a daily basis. Although specific phobias can develop at any time during life, they tend to begin during childhood and disappear with time, with or without treatment. However, treatment is helpful particularly in cases that are severe. The most common phobias are animals (dogs, snakes, spiders), heights, closed spaces (e.g., elevators), airplanes, and blood.

WHAT IS SOCIAL PHOBIA?

Social phobia, sometimes called *social anxiety,* is an intense, persistent, irrational fear that occurs when a child is around other people. Some children are afraid of specific social situations, such as speaking in public, using public restrooms, or eating in public, whereas other children might be generally afraid of most social situations. The onset of social phobia is usually during adolescence when social awareness and interactions with others become important in a child's life. To be diagnosed with a social phobia, the fear must involve avoiding situations to the point that this avoidance significantly interferes with the child's normal development.

Denise, an attractive 14-year-old high school freshman, spent much of her school day in the guidance counselor's or nurse's office. On some days, Denise would refuse to attend school, but on the days she did attend school, she had difficulty staying in the classroom. It was particularly difficult for her to stay in classes where she was expected to participate in discussions. French class was torture for her because she was expected to carry on conversations in French. When I met with Denise, she admitted that she was quite shy, even around children she knew well. She spent much time worrying about what other children thought of her and whether other children liked her. Sometimes she thought other kids were making fun of her, even when they weren't. As a very young child Denise had difficulty separating from her mom, and her mom described her as "always scared of everything." She needed constant reassurance but otherwise wasn't very anxious, except when she was around other people. That meant that she missed out on most school and recreational activities. She did not belong to clubs and rarely attended any type of party. What made Denise's case particularly sad was that her mother also was fearful of meeting new people and was content to spend much of her life in the house, often alone with Denise.

As is common with most anxiety disorders, children with social phobia usually meet criteria for other anxiety disorders as well. At different points in her development, Denise met criteria for SAD, school refusal, and *selective mutism*. By fifth grade, when Denise was required to speak in class, engage in group activities, and perform in front of others in music and gym class, she began to exhibit symptoms of social phobia. As she entered adolescence, these fears became more severe and began to have an evaluative component— Denise started to feel bad and ashamed about her symptoms and to feel she would never be normal. Denise's case was a difficult one to treat; she needed a combination of cognitive behavior therapy, school support, and medication before she could start attending school regularly and participating in class. Eventually, with the support of therapy, she began to attend some social events and was planning on attending college away from home.

Selective Mutism

When Denise (described previously) was in kindergarten, she never said a word to anyone in school. Although she talked quite freely at home with her parents, she rarely talked in any social situation, including school. She was diagnosed with *selective mutism*, a disorder in which children do not talk in specific social situations despite being quite verbal in other situations. Children with selective mutism usually show these symptoms before the age of 5 years. Some researchers feel that selective mutism might be a severe form of social phobia, and there is support for the idea that these children are more socially anxious than children with social phobia who do not exhibit this tendency. By second grade, Denise was speaking to her peers and teachers, although she was quite soft-spoken. However, as described previously, her symptoms of anxiety did not go away, they just manifested themselves in a different form.

WHAT IS OBSESSIVE–COMPULSIVE DISORDER?

Obsessions are thoughts that cannot be stopped, are unwanted, and are repetitive, whereas *compulsions* are repetitive behaviors that a child feels compelled to perform. OCD involves either obsessions or compulsions or (most often) a combination of the two. The criteria of obsession used by the American Psychiatric Association require that these obsessive thoughts

- cause the child anxiety or distress,
- are not just due to excessive "real-life" worries,
- are recognized as being a product of the child's own mind, and
- are something that the child attempts to ignore or suppress.

In terms of compulsions, the American Psychiatric Association definition requires that these repetitive behaviors are

- something that the child feels driven to perform, and
- unrealistic attempts to prevent or reduce stress or a dreaded situation.

Other criteria for OCD require that these obsessions or compulsions are very time-consuming and interfere with normal routines, family functioning, academic performance, or social relationships.

Barb was a 14-year-old high school freshman who was described by her mother as a "nervous kid." Although Barb always had friends, the stress of entering high school made her extremely nervous. She obsessed over what she was going to wear to school the next day to the point of sometimes being unable to sleep because she could not decide on the "right" outfit. She also developed a compulsion to almost constantly wash her hands. Using someone else's pencil, touching someone else's notebook, or sitting at another person's desk were all things that made her feel dirty, and she began to spend more and more time in the bathroom washing her hands. She started to be very picky about the types of foods she ate. She would only eat certain types of foods that were prepackaged, and if she opened the food and it touched the table, she refused to eat it. By the middle of her freshman year, Barb's friends started to think she was odd. Her hands were always chapped; she spent an unusual amount of time in the bathroom; and she would rarely eat around other people. Barb's school guidance counselor recommended she get treatment for her symptoms, and he consequently referred her to one of my colleagues.

Barb's presentation is not unusual. The most common obsession for children and adolescents is a concern with dirt or germs, whereas the most common compulsion is excessive hand washing, showering, or grooming. Barb had both. Other frequently observed obsessions in children include an obsession that something awful will happen, an intense need for symmetry, and a tendency to doubt whether they are right about things (e.g., "Did I do well on the test?"

Tourette's syndrome. OCD sometimes occurs with *Tourette's syndrome*, a disorder in which children display motor and vocal *tics*. Tics are sudden, recurrent motor movements or vocalizations. Motor tics can take many forms, such as eye blinking or repetitive hand movements, whereas vocal tics can take the form of a repetitive cough or blurting out certain words.

"Did I turn off the stove?"). Other frequently observed compulsions include having to repeat certain rituals; counting; or obsessively checking things such as doors, locks, or homework assignments. Barb's parents followed through with her guidance counselor's suggestion for treatment, and she received both medication and behavior therapy. OCD often follows a waxing and waning course in which symptoms emerge and fade over time; similar to many children with OCD, Barb's symptoms resurfaced when it was time for her to attend college. This time, however, she knew it was important to seek treatment again.

WHAT IS POSTTRAUMATIC STRESS DISORDER?

PTSD is an anxiety disorder that is characterized by frightening thoughts, mood disturbances, and increased feelings of physical and emotional arousal that occur after a child has been exposed to a traumatic event. Unfortunately, there is not much research on PTSD in children despite the fact that children experience high rates of chronic stress from such events as physical and sexual abuse and/or family and neighborhood violence as well as traumatic single events such as car accidents or natural disasters. PTSD can also occur in children who have experienced a direct traumatic event or witnessed a traumatic event. The triggering events usually involve an actual or threatened death or serious injury, and the child's reaction to the event must involve intense fear, feelings of hopelessness, and disorganized or agitated behavior. The symptoms that result from these feelings include continually "reliving" the trauma through intrusive thoughts, recurrent dreams, flashbacks, or psychological distress when the child is exposed to things in the environment that remind him of the trauma. Because these symptoms are so painful, the child will try to avoid feeling these feelings, and may feel "numb" or alienated from other people. In addition, the child with PTSD will display at least two or more of the following symptoms:

- trouble sleeping,
- irritability or angry outbursts,
- trouble concentrating,
- hypervigilance, and
- a tendency to startle over the slightest thing.

Some children who have experienced sexual abuse go on to develop symptoms of PTSD. This was the case with Meg, a 14-year-old who had been sexually abused by her father since the age of 6 or 7. The abuse occurred regularly until Meg disclosed to a boyfriend what her father had done. Her boyfriend told another adult, and child protective services became involved in the case. At that point, Meg was brought to the clinic for an evaluation. She was found to have mild depression and anxiety and significant symptoms related to the abuse, such as intrusive memories of the abuse, nightmares, and feelings of intense anxiety when confronted with reminders of the abuse. Meg received treatment for her symptoms. The treatment included educating her about sexual abuse (correcting misconceptions), providing her with coping skills for her symptoms of anxiety, and providing her mother with individual therapy. These cases can be quite difficult for many reasons; in the case of abuse, there is the addition of criminal charges against the abuser that can make it feel to the victim that the trauma will "never go away." Because Meg's father was subject to criminal proceedings, treatment addressed these issues as well.

ASSESSING ANXIETY DISORDERS

Formal testing is not typically used to diagnose anxiety disorders. Instead, anxiety disorders are diagnosed by interviewing the child and parents or caretakers. Regardless of the type of anxiety disorder, children who experience anxiety tend to display traits such as

- avoiding certain situations;
- crying frequently;
- refusing to go to school or to participate in school activities;
- difficulty concentrating;
- feelings of restlessness; and
- physical symptoms such as headaches, muscle pains, and stomachaches.

The evaluator will certainly ask the child and parent about these symptoms. Young children do not always understand what anxiety means, so when I interview young children, I will ask questions such as "Do you feel scared sometimes?" and "What sort of things frighten you?" I will also ask questions about whether the child feels dizzy, sweats easily, has trouble breathing, or worries about getting sick or dying. Assessing obsessions and compulsions can be particularly tricky because neither adults nor children are likely to mention these spontaneously because feelings of shame about these acts are common. It is typical that during the course of an assessment for an anxiety disorder the evaluator will have the child and parents fill out questionnaires, such as the Revised Child's Manifest Anxiety Scale or the Social Anxiety Scales for children and adolescents. The best evaluation of a child will vary depending on the child's symptoms, but using direct interviewing and questionnaires are the most typical methods.

TREATMENT OF ANXIETY DISORDERS

Treatment of anxiety disorders generally falls in two domains: psychological treatment using behavioral or cognitive behavior techniques and medication. Psychological treatments include relaxation and desensitization training, modeling, contingency management, and cognitive behavior treatment programs. *Relaxation training* teaches the child to be aware of what his body is doing when he is anxious and then provides the child with skills to control his reactions. In this type of therapy, the therapist will have the child tense and relax various muscle groups so that he can learn what tension feels like and then learn to use that feeling as a signal to relax. If a child learns to do this when he is not stressed, he can then use this strategy when he is feeling stressed. Sometimes relaxation training is combined with *desensitization training* in which the child is asked to visualize different fearful scenarios, starting with the least fearful and working up to the most feared. These visualizations are practiced while the child is in a relaxed state. This process is repeated until the child can imagine the most feared situation while staying completely relaxed.

Another psychological treatment is *modeling*. In modeling, the child observes another person interacting appropriately in a feared situation. The model can be live or on film. Sometimes the child will watch someone model the appropriate behavior and then gradually join in. For example, Jamie was a 7-year-old girl who was so afraid of spiders that she would not leave the house or classroom during the spring and summer for fear she would encounter a spider. Her psychologist first made a hierarchy of her spider fears, ranging from imagining mild fears (she might see a spider) to significant fears (actually touching one). They spent quite a bit of time working on relaxation responses to Jamie's fears, but once she could stay relaxed while imagining touching a spider, her therapist actually had her look at a real spider in a cage, then observe her therapist touching the spider, and finally touch the spider herself. Through this systematic approach, Jamie conquered her fear of spiders, and a year after her treatment, Jamie continued to have no fear.

Contingency management is a fancy way of saying that there are reinforcers when a child engages with the feared object or situation but not when she avoids it. Sometimes this treatment is referred to as *reinforced practice* in that the child is reinforced for practicing the feared behavior. Many times this is used in conjunction with modeling, relaxation, or desensitization techniques. So, for example, Jamie (mentioned previously) was given prizes each time she came closer to touching the spider.

Cognitive behavior treatments have been shown to be quite effective in treating anxiety. These treatments use a variety of strategies (such as those described earlier) to help the child recognize when she is anxious, identify what she is thinking about when she is anxious, and find skills and strategies to cope with the anxiety. The therapy might occur individually, in a group, or within a family therapy context. It may include educating children about their emotions, modeling appropriate behaviors, exposing children to the anxiety-provoking situations, role-playing, contingency rewards, teaching awareness of bodily reactions and thoughts when anxious, and relaxation techniques.

Medication can be useful in treating anxiety. The most common medications for children include selective serotonin reuptake inhibitors, tricyclic antidepressants, and antianxiety medications. Medication to treat anxiety in children is not well studied, and although it can be quite effective, it is usually not the treatment of first choice. In addition, it is likely to be used as an adjunct to psychological treatments. However, there is strong support for using selective serotonin reuptake inhibitors such as Prozac, Zoloft, Paxil, and Luvox in children with OCD. In addition, it is not unusual for psychiatrists to use a combination of medications to treat anxiety disorders, such as combining Ativan (an antianxiety medication that is taken periodically as need) with Paxil (a selective serotonin reuptake inhibitor that is taken daily). Furthermore, because anxiety disorders tend to wax and wane depending on the level of stress a child is undergoing, some children may only need medications at different times, such as the start of the school year or during stressful periods.

CONCLUDING THOUGHTS

Anxiety disorders affect up to 15% of children at some point in their development, so they are a common problem. Most children will meet criteria for more than one disorder at a time, but overall, the symptoms of anxiety tend to cluster around feelings of excessive and irrational fears. These fears are not just normal worries; they last longer than 6 months and without treatment tend to become chronic conditions.

There are a number of treatments for anxiety disorders, and most are quite effective. Various psychotherapy approaches can be used in conjunction with medication. Anxiety can be debilitating, and it is important to seek treatment if your child's symptoms are impairing his or her functioning. Left untreated, anxiety can feel overwhelming, but with the right psychological treatment, these problems can be overcome.

CHAPTER 8

LEARNING DISABILITIES

The term *learning disability* generally refers to problems in an area of learning, most specifically reading, writing, or math. The official titles of these diagnoses (according to the criteria of the *Diagnostic and Statistical Manual of Mental Disorders,* 4th ed., text rev.; American Psychiatric Association, 2000) are *reading disorder, disorder of written expression,* and *math disorder,* but you might hear the terms *dyslexia, dysgraphia,* and *dyscalculia* used instead. Of the three, reading disorder, or dyslexia, is by far the most common. Generally, to receive a diagnosis of a learning disability, a child must have a discrepancy between his intellectual ability (usually as measured on an intelligence test) and academic achievement in one or more areas. In other words, the child's performance in reading, math, or spelling is below what one would expect from him on the basis of his intellectual capabilities. Problems in one or more of these academic areas must interfere significantly with the child's ability to perform in school. The problem also cannot be due to a lack of instruction because a child who has not been taught to read (and therefore cannot read) does not have a reading disability; his problem with reading is due to poor instruction. Similarly, the problem with learning academics cannot be due to problems with cognitive skills because a child who is diagnosed with mental retardation would be expected to have difficulties learning academics.

WHAT IS DYSLEXIA?

Kevin was an enthusiastic second grader who loved everything about school—except for reading. He was the first one to answer any math question, popular with the kids in his class, and great on the soccer field. However, homework time, according to his mom, was a "nightmare." He cried when he had to write 10 sentences using his spelling words and didn't like going to school on Fridays because it was "spelling test day." In preschool and kindergarten Kevin had difficulty learning his letters and had trouble sounding out words. His first- and second-grade teachers had told his parents, "He's a boy and a late bloomer, don't worry." However, now it was the end of second grade, and Kevin's parents were worried because he still could not read any of his assignments without great struggle. His father was particularly worried because he himself struggled with reading as a child and never went to college because school was so difficult for him. He didn't want to see the same thing happen to his son.

Kevin was eventually diagnosed with dyslexia. Children with dyslexia, or reading disorder, have a problem accurately and fluently reading words. Recent research has demonstrated that *phonological processing* is the underlying problem in most cases of reading disorders; phonological processing includes the skills involved in understanding the rules by which sounds go with letters. This is sometimes referred to as *letter–sound correspondence*. For instance, children must learn that dog has three sounds (or *phonemes)* in it. First, they have to be able to hear and segment these sounds; then they have to blend the sounds together to form the word. Children with dyslexia have difficulty perceiving the individual sounds or phonemes in words and, therefore, have trouble with the task of breaking words down to sound them out for reading or spelling.

Many parents think that dyslexia means that children reverse letters or write backward. Although some children with dyslexia do have a tendency to reverse letters, this is not the defining feature of the disorder. In addition, although many children with dyslexia dislike reading, some actually do like to read, and a fair number have good reading comprehension (i.e., understanding what they have read). However, by definition, nearly all children with dyslexia have difficulty learning phonics and have trouble with reading fluency. It's a struggle for them to sound out words they have not seen before, and spelling can be quite difficult. Because dyslexia is a language-based learning disability (reading is a language task), many children with dyslexia have difficulty with other aspects of language, such as problems with verbal memory, word-finding difficulties, or difficulty organizing their thoughts. Problems with writing are quite common as well.

Most children with dyslexia do not have problems in their early history, such as prenatal or birth traumas, and they do not typically have problems reaching normal developmental milestones, such as walking. However, some do have articulation problems (i.e., problems pronouncing words) or speech delays in early childhood. By first or second grade, children with dyslexia are typically showing problems with reading. In fact, their problems might be evident as early as kindergarten in that they may have difficulty learning the alphabet or letter sounds. Research has shown a strong family risk factor in dyslexia in that it seems to run in families. In other words, there is a strong genetic component to dyslexia.

HOW IS DYSLEXIA ASSESSED?

An evaluation for dyslexia needs to be tailored to the individual child so that it reflects the child's age and level of education. For example, an evaluation for a first grader who is having difficulty learning to read will be very different from an evaluation for a ninth grader. In any case, the evaluation needs to establish that there is a reading problem by evaluating reading decoding skills and comprehension skills. At an earlier age, the ability to read accurately is typically impaired in children with dyslexia, but as children age and receive treatment, they may learn to read accurately, if more slowly. Thus, a dyslexia evaluation needs to include the following components, which need to be geared to the child's educational and developmental level:

- Tests of decoding: A reading evaluation needs to determine how accurately a child can decode words.
- Tests of reading nonsense words: The ability to read nonsense words is the best measure of phonological processing skills in children, and all evaluations for dyslexia should in include a test of nonsense words (sometimes called *pseudowords*). On these tests, children are asked to read words they have never seen before, such as vip, ziptum, or lightmum. Because children have never seen these words before (and have not just memorized the word), the only way they can sound these words out is to use decoding, or phonics, skills.
- Tests of reading comprehension: These tests assess the child's ability to understand what he has read. However, sometimes children with dyslexia can do quite well on tests of reading comprehension because they are good at inferring the meaning of the passage, even if they have not read the entire passage correctly.
- Tests of oral reading: Tests of oral reading are good measures of a child's reading fluency. During the evaluation, the assessor will also be listening for qualitative errors that the child might display, such as a slow reading, problems pronouncing words, and a lack of cadence in the reading.

In addition to these areas, children with dyslexia have difficulty with spelling and written expression, and a comprehensive evaluation

Language-Based Learning Disabilities

Sometimes the term *language-based learning disability* is used interchangeably with dyslexia, but they actually are two different disorders. In dyslexia, the major problem is in phonological processing, and the child's language system is primarily intact. In a language-based learning disability, the major problem involves all aspects of language, which often includes both the sounds and the meanings of words. The reading difficulties can occur at both the decoding and comprehension levels, and various language difficulties are observed.

needs to explore these areas. Finally, a comprehensive evaluation needs to include a measure of intellectual abilities and measures of general language functioning. Because as many as 24% of children with dyslexia will also have attention-deficit/hyperactivity disorder (ADHD), it is important to rule out the possibility of ADHD through the use of observations, behavior rating scales, and screening for problems with executive function skills.

It is important to note that no single test can provide a diagnosis of dyslexia. The diagnosis can be made only after a comprehensive battery of tests has been provided by a qualified psychologist. At a minimum, a core battery needs to include a measure of cognitive skills, reading (accuracy, fluency, and comprehension), spelling, and general language. It is the overall pattern that is important, and this pattern can look very different depending on the child.

For example, Polly was a very bright 8-year-old child whose reading skills were in the average range; however, she had significant difficulty with decoding unfamiliar words, and as she progressed in school, her reading fluency began to suffer more and more. Even though some of her reading skills were within the average range, she was not performing at her above-average expectations on specific areas of functioning, which indicated a diagnosis of dyslexia. She was keeping up with her peers (although just barely), but she was not keeping up with her potential, and as she matured it became harder for her to keep up with her peers as well. Billy, on the other hand, was an 8-year-old boy with low-average cognitive skills whose reading levels were far below grade and cognitive expectations. Without very significant intervention, there was a possibility that Billy could be illiterate. Although both children had dyslexia, Billy's difficulties were more severe.

WHAT ARE THE BEST TREATMENTS FOR DYSLEXIA?

Fortunately, there are a number of proven methods for remediating dyslexia. Some of the more popular approaches are the Orton-Gillingham, Wilson Reading System, and Lindamood Bell. These programs are meant to be administered in small groups or one-to-one settings and have a few things in common. They are *multisensory* in their approach (using many senses, such as visual cues, touch, verbal skills); they are *sequential* in that each skill builds on another one; and they are *phonologically based* (use phonics to teach reading). There are also a few programs that have been developed for children who have early signs of reading problems, with the most popular approach being the Reading Mastery approach. Although each of these programs emphasizes different aspects of reading, research has indicated that each of these methods is as good as the other as long as they are implemented by well-trained tutors with sufficient intensity (frequently enough to make a difference) and for a sufficient duration (in other words, not stopping tutoring too soon).

Although phonological processing is the major difficulty that needs to be remediated in children with dyslexia, most children also need support in reading fluency. Daily practicing of oral reading (even for short amounts of time, such as 5 or 10 minutes) can help, and programs such as ReadIt use speech recognition technology to improve reading fluency in children from Grades 2 through 5. One of most important things that parents can do is to read to their children and to have their children read aloud to them. This is frequently not a fun task for most children with dyslexia, so having children read passages that are easy for them or read fun poetry, such as Dr. Seuss or Shel Silverstein, can be a way of making this task less laborious.

Finally, Dr. Sally Shaywitz, one of the leading researchers on dyslexia, has identified several components of a successful reading intervention. First, the earlier the intervention begins, the better the outcome. Second, the intervention needs to be intensive enough that it makes a difference. Many times, this means getting tutoring in a very small group (no more than two other children) four to five times per week. Third, the tutoring needs to be high quality. Although this might seem obvious, it is a quite common occurrence for children to receive tutoring from a classroom aide or an unqualified teacher. However, research indicates that children show the most progress when they have skilled tutors. Thus, advocating for an experienced, well-trained tutor is essential. Finally, the treatment needs to occur for a sufficient duration—in other words, treatment should not end prematurely. Within the public school setting, it is not unusual for a child's services to be limited prematurely as a result of budget constraints. However, these skills need to be *overlearned,* and taking away services prematurely can undermine much of the achieved progress. Thus, it is important for parents to be familiar with their child's reading progress and service delivery. Finally, monitoring a child's performance through regular evaluations (either through a private-practice psychologist or the school system) is an important way to make sure the services are working.

WHAT IS MATH DISORDER?

A math disorder can be diagnosed when there is a discrepancy between a child's math computation skills or math reasoning skills and his or her aptitude or cognitive skills. Math disorder occurs in about 6% of children, and there are no known causes. This can be a difficult issue to diagnose because poor performance in math can also be due to performance anxiety and motivation, and math problems often co-occur with other learning disabilities, such as ADHD, dyslexia, expressive and receptive language disorders, and nonverbal learning disabilities (NLDs).

A math disorder cannot be diagnosed until a child has had formal math instruction. Although there are a number of mathematical concepts and skills that preschoolers naturally acquire through the environment, it is not until elementary school that mastery of concepts and written calculations is required. Unfortunately, there is not one special skill that is impaired in children with a math disorder (as phonological processing is in dyslexia). Instead, children with a math disorder tend to have vulnerabilities in a number of different areas, such as visual–motor skills (writing and copying numbers), fact mastery (memorizing times tables), memorization of math formulas, following multistep directions, understanding higher level abstract language skills that are needed for solving complex story problems, and reasoning and abstract logic abilities. There is no "typical" child with a math disability, and by the time these children are diagnosed, they may be anxious about—and dislike—math.

Molly was a ninth-grade student who had been struggling with math since second grade. It was never too much of an issue because Molly was a good reader and a dedicated student. However, as the math concepts became more difficult, she started to develop a fear of anything that was related to math. Her problems with math started to interfere with other subjects, especially science, and she was failing freshman chemistry. She started to become anxious about all tests, not just those that involved math, and when her parents brought her in for an evaluation, they were afraid that she would not graduate from high school. Her mother felt guilty as she admitted that she was "bad at math" too, but she had been afraid to have Molly tested for fear that they would find something "really wrong."

Molly's story is quite common, as children with math problems don't tend to be identified early in their academic careers. It's often not until the problems with math cause another problem (such as test anxiety or poor performance in math or multiple subjects) that a child is assessed. A full neuropsychological evaluation indicated that Molly had problems in a number of areas related to math: she had difficulty with *short-term memory* in that despite years of drilling and memorizing math facts, she still did not know her times tables. She had problems remembering the steps, or procedures, needed to complete complex math problems such as algebraic formulae or long division. Finally, she had *visuospatial deficits* that made it difficult for her to see things geometrically.

HOW IS MATH DISORDER ASSESSED?

Math disorder is typically assessed through the use of a comprehensive test battery, such as the test battery that is used in a neuropsychological evaluation. The evaluator must look at a number of different aspects of math achievement, such as *computational arithmetic* and *conceptual understanding of math* (i.e., applying math concepts to things such as story problems). The evaluating psychologist will also want to take a detailed history and look at the types of errors that the child has made. Having this diagnosis made in the context of a comprehensive neuropsychological evaluation is important because it can pinpoint other cognitive skill deficits that may

129

contribute to the child's learning disabilities and identify areas of strength on which to build.

WHAT ARE THE BEST TREATMENTS FOR MATH DISORDER?

Unfortunately, there are no well-validated, standardized treatment approaches for children with learning disabilities in math (as there are for children with reading disabilities). In fact, individualized programs that respond to a child's individual needs are necessary. The individualization refers to not only what the child needs to learn but also to how he or she learns. For example, some students learn best through rote drill, whereas others learn math facts by associating the facts with previously learned information. Some children have difficulty with perceptual skills, such as size relationships, distance, and sequencing, whereas other children have difficulty mentally shifting from one concept to another. Many children who have difficulty in math have trouble with abstract thinking, and most have difficulties in more than one of these areas; each area will need to be addressed in the course of remediation.

In general, the following guidelines have been found to be important in teaching children with math disabilities:

- Students need to be taught the full range of math skills, including math facts, operations, word problems, reasoning skills, time, fractions, and measurement.
- Students need to learn the language of math—the concepts such as half, percentage, or perimeter.
- If a student is not succeeding with one approach, the teaching needs to be flexible enough to make a change.
- Concrete materials and real-life applications of math help children transfer math skills to other contexts.
- Students need to have opportunities to practice these skills in many different ways.

WHAT IS DISORDER OF WRITTEN EXPRESSION?

Children with learning disabilities in writing typically have problems in handwriting, spelling, and composition. Their problems go beyond just bad penmanship to the point at which their writing is illegible. It can take them a very long time to come up with a topic, and once they do, they can be slow at the act of writing. Spelling can be a problem, and their writing can consist of short sentences that lack a theme. They typically don't use strategies such as planning out their story, organizing the story, writing a rough draft, or editing. Although writing problems are often noticed by age 8 years (the time when children are asked to do more writing in school), these problems sometimes go undiagnosed until middle or high school. By that time, the problem has taken another form in that it looks like the child or adolescent is just poorly motivated or "not trying." Furthermore, a disorder of written expression is commonly found in combination with a reading or math disorder, and many children with ADHD also struggle with writing issues.

The act of writing involves language, visual skills, and the motor skills needed to form letters. Because of this, a disorder of written expression can include some combination of fine motor problems, language problems, visual–spatial problems, and attention and memory problems. Some children may have difficulty tracing shapes or writing letters; others may be able to form letters well, but they may be very slow; still other children have good penmanship but cannot organize their thoughts well enough to write a well-formed paragraph or story. Because research on this disorder and in this area is lacking, psychologists know less about this disorder than other types of learning disabilities. It affects about 8% to 15% of school-age children, and many of these children have other learning issues as well.

HOW IS DISORDER OF WRITTEN EXPRESSION ASSESSED?

A comprehensive evaluation, such as a neuropsychological evaluation, that looks at many aspects of writing and associated skills is typically used to make a diagnosis of a disorder of written expression. Typically this includes a measure of intelligence, tests of academic achievement (with a particular emphasis on writing skills), tests of visual–motor abilities, and tests that may be needed to rule out comorbid conditions, such as ADHD. The evaluator will also make qualitative evaluations, looking at how the child writes letters or sentences. The evaluator may also ask to see samples of the child's writing from school.

For example, when I evaluated Julie, her mother brought in a folder of classroom writing assignments completed within the past year. I noticed immediately that she had made many spelling and writing errors, alternated between printing and cursive, and used simple sentence structure. Sometimes her writing was illegible. On the tests of writing that she completed with me, Julie's performance fell below the average range. She took a long time to do any paper-and-pencil tasks and exhibited slow processing speed. Her overall performance was consistent with a disorder of written expression in that she had significant problems with spelling, capitalization, punctuation, and grammar. She had difficulty with paragraph and sentence structure. Her use of complex language was quite limited, and her handwriting was very poor. I made a number of recommendations for Julie, one being that she receive further evaluation from an occu-

Occupational therapists (OTs) evaluate and treat fine motor and daily living skills (also known as *occupational skills*) in children and adults. In children with handwriting problems, OTs help them develop the fine motor and perceptual–motor abilities that contribute to good handwriting skills.

pational therapist to assess the fine motor coordination problems that seemed to be involved in Julie's writing difficulties.

WHAT ARE THE BEST TREATMENTS FOR DISORDER OF WRITTEN EXPRESSION?

Interventions for learning disabilities in writing have been developed but have not yet been well studied. Much like a math disorder, writing skills include many areas, such as formulating ideas, organizing the ideas, using correct grammar, spelling the words correctly, and writing legibly. Many treatment programs focus on just one or two of these issues. In terms of the physical ability to write legibly, occupational therapy is frequently recommended. OTs assist children in learning the mechanics of letter formation. They evaluate a child's grip and treat any associated fine motor and sensorimotor weaknesses that a child might have. One particular program, Handwriting Without Tears, is frequently used by OTs and teachers to teach handwriting to children. Other treatment programs focus on the ability to put one's thoughts in writing. Most programs teach writing as a process that includes prewriting activities (e.g., organizing and sequencing ideas), the writing itself, and postwriting activities (e.g., editing). Some programs help children organize their ideas by using prepared templates for the mapping or webbing of ideas. These are sometimes referred to as *graphic organizers*. They can come in various shapes, such as a topic wheel or a sequential outline.

In addition to teaching children the skills they need, *accommodations* to the learning environment are typically made. These can include use of a computer, assistance with note-taking (such as getting notes from a friend or teacher), allowing students to tape lectures, providing extra time for written assignments and tests, and providing opportunities to demonstrate knowledge through means other than written work. Programs such as Dragon NaturallySpeaking, in which

133

a computer prints text as the person speaks into the computer, can also be helpful.

WHAT IS A NONVERBAL LEARNING DISABILITY?

An NLD is a syndrome that includes problems in visual–spatial organization, nonverbal problem solving, and social skills. Despite often having strong verbal abilities, children with NLD have difficulty appreciating humor and have problems adapting to new situations. Academically, they generally have better reading skills than math skills, and they often have trouble with writing skills and executive functions. Problems with social judgment and social interactions are frequently considered part of this diagnosis. Although this diagnosis is frequently used, there is some disagreement as to its validity and just what this diagnosis means. There is a high degree of overlap with this disorder and Asperger's syndrome, and some experts believe these may be the same disorder viewed with different lenses. However, other professionals have argued that these are two different disorders and that NLD is a valid diagnosis.

What is known about NLD is that the deficits that these children have are multifaceted and include at least some or most of the following symptoms:

- lower nonverbal IQ scores (i.e., Perceptual Reasoning on the Wechsler Intelligence Scale for Children, 4th ed.) as compared with verbal IQ scores (i.e., Verbal Comprehension on the Wechsler Intelligence Scale for Children, 4th ed.);
- academic weaknesses in written expression, math, and/or reading comprehension;
- fine motor skills weaknesses;
- poor social skills;
- gross motor coordination weaknesses;

- problems with abstract language and pragmatic language;
- trouble getting organized;
- problems shifting from one task to another; and
- associated emotional problems such as anxiety, emotional outbursts, and withdrawal.

HOW IS NONVERBAL LEARNING DISABILITY DIAGNOSED?

Typically NLD is diagnosed through a neuropsychological evaluation by a psychologist who will evaluate all of the areas mentioned previously. The evaluation will include a measure of intelligence, academic tests, visual-spatial and visual–motor tests, language tests, tests of executive function skills, and measures of social and behavioral functioning. A full test battery can be quite helpful in distinguishing NLD from other disorders. This sort of specialized testing, which includes a formal diagnosis, is not typically provided through the school system. Although testing completed through the public schools will describe the concerns, the evaluator will not give a formal diagnosis because that is not the typical function of a school psychologist. If having a formal diagnosis and complete documentation of the child's strengths and weaknesses is important to you, you will need to get an evaluation completed by a licensed psychologist who works in private practice or in a clinic or hospital setting.

WHAT ARE THE BEST TREATMENTS FOR NONVERBAL LEARNING DISORDER?

Treatments for NLD are as varied as the symptoms themselves. For children who have trouble with motor skills, treatment by an OT is important. For those who have trouble with social language skills, speech and language therapy is typically prescribed. Physical therapy is the treatment of choice for children who have problems with gross motor coordination and strength. Other prescribed treatments include

- an appropriate classroom placement with a low student–teacher ratio;
- social skills training;
- tutoring in reading comprehension, math, writing, or executive function skills, as needed;
- psychotherapy to treat associated symptoms such as anxiety; and
- sometimes medication to treat associated problems of attention, mood, and anxiety.

LEARNING DISABILITIES: WHAT PARENTS CAN DO

Many, if not most, children with learning disabilities are quite capable of attending college and having satisfying and competitive careers—particularly if they receive appropriate treatment. Getting an appropriate diagnosis that focuses the treatment on the specific areas of need is important. Finding the right treatment resources can be difficult because there is a lack of good tutors and allied services providers in many areas of the country—but be persistent! One of the most important things parents can do is to educate themselves on their child's disability because this knowledge puts them in a much better position to advocate for their child's services. Working collaboratively with the school and service providers (while not relinquishing the role of advocate) is key. Research in the field of learning disabilities is constantly yielding advances in understanding and treating learning disabilities, and there is much reason for optimism in the diagnosis and treatment of children with a wide variety of learning issues. In Chapter 15, I discuss the role of the school in this process, including when it is appropriate to seek services from the school.

CONCLUDING THOUGHTS

Specific learning disabilities fall into three broad categories: reading disabilities, math disabilities, and writing disabilities. In addition, some children experience learning disabilities in nonverbal problem solving. There are many treatments for all of these issues, and many of these treatments can be provided through your child's school. In this case, your child's school psychologist is the best place to start. In addition, your child may need additional treatment, such as talking to a psychologist outside of school or receiving tutoring after school hours. If you suspect your child may have a learning disability, it will be important to have a thorough evaluation. You can receive this type of evaluation through your local school system or by a psychologist who works in private practice or a medical setting. Above all, the evaluation should be your first step in determining treatment. Following through with recommendations is the next step in making sure your child gets the help he or she needs.

CHAPTER 9

EATING DISORDERS

Mindy was never satisfied with her body during middle school. She would complain that she was fat and refuse to eat despite the entreaties of her mother and everyone around her. By age 15, when she arrived at her psychologist's office for the first time, she looked like a walking skeleton. She had spent the last 3 months eating nothing but carrot sticks and small bites of protein bars. Whenever she had free time, you could find her exercising in her room or at the gym. Her mother had become concerned the week before, when she went to hug Mindy and realized she was "nothing but bones." She had also noticed that Mindy's once-thick blond hair now hung in strings, and her complexion was yellow and sallow. When the psychologist asked Mindy how she thought she looked, Mindy said, "I've never looked better."

Tina never worried too much about her weight until she arrived at college at age 18 and started putting on the "freshman 15." Tina was having lots of fun at school—drinking beers at parties and eating pizza and munchies late at night—but within 5 months she had gained 15 pounds. She tried dieting and exercising, but because she continued to eat large amounts of food, especially late at night, she could not lose any weight until she started forcing herself to vomit.

This did not help Tina diminish in size, but she felt she could at least maintain her weight this way despite eating enormous amounts of cookies, candies, cake, and pizza. Tina felt ashamed of her behavior and by the end of her freshman year was depressed as well. Tina was referred to an eating disorders clinic where she became involved in group therapy and received medication to treat her depression.

Tina and Mindy have two different types of eating disorders. Mindy's symptoms are consistent with a diagnosis of anorexia (sometimes referred to as *anorexia nervosa),* whereas Tina's symptoms are consistent with bulimia (sometimes referred to as *bulimia nervosa).* These are both complicated disorders and are among the few disorders that affect mainly women, although boys and men can have these disorders as well.

WHAT IS ANOREXIA?

Anorexia is characterized by a refusal to maintain a healthy body weight, which is typically defined as 15% below normal for a child's height and weight. Most people with anorexia feel just as Mindy does: They think they look great when they are at their thinnest and often are unsatisfied with the low bodyweight they achieve. In fact, they will think they look fat even though they are actually frail and very thin. Girls with anorexia fail to have menstrual periods. Even though they restrict their food intake, they are typically obsessed with food. For example, Mindy's favorite shows were cooking shows, and she often enjoyed cooking the family dinner, even if she never ate a bite. In her free time she could be found reading cookbooks or exercising. Despite her obsession with food, she ate very little and would obsessively control her caloric intake—sometimes only eating 400 calories a day.

There are two types of anorexia, the *restricting* type and the *binge-eating and purging* type. Mindy has the restricting type because her symptoms include the following:

- refusing to maintain a normal body weight,
- an intense fear of gaining weight, and
- a distorted way of thinking about her body in that she experiences her size as much larger than it actually is.

Young people with restricting anorexia tend to achieve their weight loss by fasting and/or excessively exercising. In the binge-eating and purging type, the child or adolescent engages in regular episodes of bingeing (overeating to the extreme) or purging (vomiting after overeating). This is not the same type of pattern as bulimia (described later) because compared with young people with bulimia (who tend to eat large quantities of food before purging), young people with the binge-eating and purging type of anorexia tend to eat small amounts of food and subsequently purge more consistently and thoroughly.

Anorexia typically develops during adolescence, with peaks at ages 14 and 18. Children who have not yet reached adolescence can be diagnosed with anorexia, but it is rare. Some adolescents just experience one episode of anorexia, while others "yo-yo" between periods of fairly normal weight and underweight. Anorexia is a very serious condition because extreme weight loss can lead to a number of significant medical complications, such as heart problems, dental problems, loss of bone density, anemia, hair loss, and hormonal changes. The disorder can be life threatening, and some statistics indicate that up to 10% of cases of individuals with anorexia end in death, although half of those cases may result from suicide.

Possible Signs of Anorexia

- extreme thinness, almost skeleton-like;
- acting "funny" around food—does not want to eat around family members, plays with food, acts like a "picky eater," will only eat unusual food combinations;
- wearing loose-fitting, baggy clothing;
- osteoporosis;
- anxious energy;
- skipping meals (and gives a "good" excuse for skipping meals);
- constipation;
- mood problems such as depressed mood, irritability, moodiness, and withdrawal; and
- intolerance to cold.

WHAT IS BULIMIA?

Remember Tina at the beginning of this chapter? She had bulimia. Bulimia usually develops a little later than anorexia and can develop from anorexia. It often begins during the college years, when the desire to be thin and attractive to the opposite sex becomes increasingly important. Tina exhibits all of the classic features of bulimia, which include the following:

- frequent episodes of binge eating, which is rapidly eating large amounts of food—larger amounts than most people would eat in a typical situation (i.e., a gallon of ice cream and/or two bags of cookies)—and a lack of control of this type of eating;
- attempts to prevent weight gain after bingeing, which can include vomiting, using medications such as diuretics or laxatives, fasting, or excessively exercising;
- binge eating and subsequent attempts to prevent weight loss that occur at least twice a week for 3 months; and

- a self-perception that is distorted in terms of body shape and weight.

There are two types of bulimia. Tina had the *purging* type in that she typically vomited (purged) or used laxatives to control her weight. The other type of bulimia is the *nonpurging* type in which the typical behaviors used to control weight are fasting or excessive exercising. Most individuals diagnosed with bulimia (almost 90%) engage in self-induced vomiting.

Individuals with bulimia tend to be very ashamed of their problem—much more so than those with anorexia. In fact, adolescents with bulimia tend to feel very bad about themselves after bingeing, and they tend to hide their problem from their friends and family. A typical binge can be over 5,000 calories and even much more than that. I have heard adolescents with bulimia admit to baking two dozen cinnamon rolls and eating every one. They may eat two pizzas followed by two pints of ice cream. This type of eating can be very costly, and some children and adolescents with bulimia will steal food. Bingeing is typically done in private; for example, when a roommate is gone for the night or the parents are already asleep. Most people with bulimia aren't aware that they are already full, and they will continue to eat until they are "found out," fall asleep, have stomach pain, or induce vomiting. Sometimes inducing vomiting will allow them to continue to binge. After a binge, most people experience feelings of guilt and sadness.

Bulimia is a very serious disorder, although most patients with bulimia make a complete recovery. It is less dangerous than anorexia (death is rare), but there are significant health problems associated with this disorder. These problems include edema (i.e., swelling of the hands and feet), stomach pains, dental problems as a result of loss of enamel, menstrual irregularities, dehydration, and heart problems. It may surprise you to hear that many individuals with binge-eating

---

Possible Signs of Bulimia

- binge eating;
- frequent trips to the bathroom, especially after a large meal or binge eating;
- mood problems, such as depression, irritability, and fatigue;
- dental problems, particularly erosion of the enamel and gum disease;
- gastrointestinal problems, such as constipation, bloating, diarrhea (from the use of laxatives), and abdominal pain;
- frequent weigh fluctuation; and
- secretive eating and dislike of eating in front of others.

---

problems are overweight and sometimes obese. Even though they try to control their weight through purging and the use of laxatives, their caloric intake is so high that they gain weight in spite of their efforts to the contrary.

WHAT CAUSES EATING DISORDERS?

Many individuals with eating disorders tend be the "perfect" child before developing symptoms. In addition to the symptoms indicated previously, adolescents with eating disorders tend to be perfectionistic, need to be in control, and have a distorted perception of their bodies. Some theorists have suggested that anorexia is caused in part by a culture that has an incredibly absurd ideal of thinness, especially for women. The pressure to look like the "ideal" woman who is represented on the covers of magazines drives many women to diet. In adolescence this pressure is combined with the fact that adolescents have to develop their own identities, individuate from their families, become comfortable with their sexuality, and be accepted by their peers. Some adolescents are more susceptible to these pressures, particularly those who have low self-esteem, are overcontrolling and rigid, and grow up in families in which problems don't typically get resolved openly. These theories have yet to be completely proven. However, biological theories of eating disorders do have some research support. Many researchers believe that there are multiple genes for eating disorders and that these genes combine with environmental factors to increase a person's susceptibility to develop an eating disorder.

Other factors that have been identified with eating disorders include early feeding difficulties in that picky eating and digestive problems in early childhood increase the risk of developing anorexia in adolescence. Although more research is needed to clarify this connection, it does appear that experiences in early childhood regarding food patterns and control over what one is allowed to eat are factors in shaping later eating problems. Similarly, the family's and the child's weight history are considered possible factors in the development of eating disorders. For example, extreme weight concerns, a family history of obesity, and a history of childhood obesity are associated with developing eating disorders. Finally, early sexual abuse has been shown to be a risk factor for eating-disordered behavior, although the nature of this relationship is unclear. There is no single cause of anorexia. Its causes are complex and most likely a combination of social, biological, and environmental factors.

HOW ARE ANOREXIA AND BULIMIA ASSESSED?

Anorexia and bulimia are complex disorders, and because of this a *multimodal* assessment process is needed. A multimodal process means that different professionals are used to make an appropriate assessment. This team usually includes a psychologist or mental health professional, psychiatrist or medical doctor, and a nutritionist. A good assessment will not only evaluate the potential for eating disorders but will also evaluate other psychological disorders that frequently cooccur with eating disorders, such as depression, anxiety, obsessive–compulsive disorder, and substance use disorders. Don't be surprised if a large part of the evaluation process is devoted to assessing the family environment. This is especially true if the patient is younger than 18 years of age and still living at home. The evaluator will probably want to evaluate family variables such as

- the parents' perception about when and how the eating disorder began,
- the parents' thoughts on why the eating disorder occurred,
- the types of changes the parents have seen in their child's behavior since the eating disorder began,
- the child's developmental history,
- any type of family difficulties or stressors that have occurred during the child's development,
- the impact of the family on the child's eating disorder, and
- the parents' knowledge and expectations regarding the process of becoming an adolescent and what that may mean to the family's functioning.

In addition to assessing the family's functioning, the evaluator will also want to look at the child's interpersonal, social, and environmental functioning. Studies have shown that many individuals with eating disorders have interpersonal difficulties. Some (about 20% to 30%) are excessively shy or have a history of difficulty making close friends. For those who did not have difficulty making friends before their eating disorder, the eating disorder itself can interfere a great deal with social relationships or school performance because peers find the obsession with food off-putting or strange or the child is so physically exhausted by the lack of adequate nutrition that she does not typically have the mental energy for academics or social relationships. Thus, it is important for the evaluator to look at all of these variables.

Finally, it is crucial for patients with eating disorders to undergo a thorough medical assessment. A typical medical evaluation will include

- a physical examination;
- laboratory tests;
- blood counts;
- urine analysis; and
- a review of major body systems, such as the heart and cardio-vascular, lungs, eyes, gastrointestinal, and musculoskeletal.

The medical doctor will want to know if the child experiences weakness, tiredness, constipation, or depression because these can be due to electrolyte disturbances that can occur from excessive vomiting or laxative use.

Can Guys Have Eating Disorders?

The answer to this question is yes, and it's possible that eating disorders in males are more common than one might expect. However, although men with eating disorder tend to show the same symptoms as women (i.e., preoccupation with food, negative body image), they tend to place less of an emphasis on a drive for thinness and more of an emphasis on athletic appearance, although they may become quite thin in the process. They may also engage in bulimic behaviors to stay a certain weight for a sport such as wrestling or boxing. It's quite possible that the increased pictures that are seen in advertisements of the male physique with the "six-pack abs" can be contributing to disordered eating, harmful weight control, or unhealthy or obsessive body-building behaviors in males.

WHAT ARE THE TREATMENTS FOR EATING DISORDERS?

The major treatments for eating disorders include family therapy, cognitive behavior therapy (CBT), interpersonal psychotherapy, and medication. Group therapy is also often helpful. Because eating disorders are complex and are caused by multiple factors, treatments need to address multiple influences. It is crucial to work with a treatment team that specializes in eating disorders. The treatment team typically includes a psychologist, primary care physician, psychopharmacologist (if medication is prescribed), and a nutritionist. It is important to find professionals who have a wealth of experience treating eating disorders because these disorders can be difficult to treat. Unfortunately, even though these treatments are widely used, the evidence for their effectiveness is somewhat limited, especially for anorexia. In other words, eating disorders are difficult to treat, and much remains to be learned about how best to treat them.

Family Therapy

Family therapy is often the initial treatment of choice for children and adolescents who are still living at home. The therapist will spend time helping the family develop health-communication skills. He or she will assess the family's attitudes toward food and body image. Family therapy does not necessarily mean that the whole family will attend every therapy session. Sometimes the therapist will meet separately with the child and the parents. Remember Mindy from the beginning of this chapter? In the course of family therapy, Mindy's parents admitted they had difficulty taking control over Mindy's eating patterns, telling their therapist, Mindy always "did whatever she wanted to do with her food—even as a toddler!" The therapist used her time with Mindy's parents to help them establish control within the family system. She spent time educating the parents on the developmental tasks of adolescence and gave them hope. She made sure the treatment focused on

Mindy's illness, not on placing blame on particular family members. Mindy's father was prone to saying to his wife, "You always let her do what she wanted, and that's why we're in this mess," but throughout the course of therapy, the therapist challenged these statements and helped the parents build an alliance between the two of them and with Mindy.

Cognitive Behavior Therapy

CBT has been shown to be particularly effective for bulimia but is a treatment of choice for anorexia as well. Cognitive behavior therapists change eating patterns by rewarding or modeling "good" behaviors. Within this approach, the therapist will challenge the patient's belief system. For example, Mindy (whose therapist used a combination of family therapy and CBT) felt she was "fat" even though she was 5'4" and weighed 95 pounds. The therapist helped Mindy modify her thinking about normal body weight and shape by having her examine her views about the "ideal" woman. She helped Mindy replace her dieting and purging with more normal eating habits through having her monitor her food intake and bingeing and purging episodes. She then explored with Mindy the thoughts and feelings that seemed to trigger these episodes. Mindy was weighed frequently during her sessions, and she was encouraged to eat foods she was avoiding and to plan out her meals. Through the course of therapy (which lasted almost 2 years), Mindy and her therapist constantly reviewed what was working and what was not working, and this helped Mindy avoid relapsing into her old habits.

Interpersonal Psychotherapy

Interpersonal therapy has been shown to be quite beneficial in treating bulimia, especially if the treatment is long term. Although research data have not shown support for the effectiveness of this approach in treating anorexia, it is sometimes used in conjunction with other approaches in treating anorexia. Interpersonal therapy addresses the interpersonal—situational and personal—issues that contribute to the development and maintenance of the disorder. This treatment has been found to be as effective as CBT in treating eating disorders, but it tends to work somewhat more slowly. Some experts have suggested that interpersonal therapy may address issues such as problems with social relationships, negative emotions, and low self-esteem, and that addressing these issues helps to break the maladaptive behaviors associated with eating disorders. Interpersonal therapy does not directly target a person's eating symptoms but instead focuses on one or more

Interpersonal Therapy Problem Areas

Grief. Therapy may target unresolved grief that could have occurred after a loss of a loved one or another significant loss, such as a divorce. The goals of treatment are to facilitate the mourning process and reestablish healthy relationships that can take the place of what was lost.

Role disputes. These types of disputes occur when the child and at least one significant other (usually one or both of the parents) have differing expectations of the relationship. Therapy will focus on helping identify the nature of the disputes and will begin to modify the patterns (sometimes using adjunctive family therapy) or change the expectations of those involved.

Role transitions. Problems with role transitions occur when a person has difficulty coping with life changes that require new roles. These problems are quite common in adolescence, particularly late adolescence, when the child is often leaving the home environment. If this is the problem, therapy will focus on adjusting to the new role by acquiring new skills and developing new social networks.

Interpersonal deficits. These problems are seen in families in which there is a history of inadequate or unsupportive personal relationships. The goal of treatment is to examine past relationships while simultaneously learning ways to form new relationships.

of four interpersonal problem areas, such as role transitions, role disputes, interpersonal deficits, and grief. Early in therapy the therapist will identify which of these four areas is most closely associated with the onset of the maladaptive eating behaviors. Because the onset of symptoms can be linked to stressful events, such as the loss of a parent, the onset of menses and adolescence, and school transitions, this therapy can be useful in addressing the underlying issues.

Samantha: Coping With Interpersonal Deficits

Samantha was a 16-year-old with bulimia who was a junior in high school and who came from a family in which inadequate personal relationships were the norm. Her parents separated when she was 11 years old, but before the separation they fought constantly; her father could be quite violent, whereas her mother could be described as a pushover. After the separation, her grandmother moved in to help take care of her and her brother. This only served to increase the tension in the house because her mother and her grandmother did not get along. Samantha's mother, Robyn, cared about her but had difficulty showing it. Robyn worked as a legal secretary at a location 40 miles from home, which meant she left the house early and came home late. In addition, she spent many nights with her boyfriend while Samantha stayed with her grandmother. When Robyn had vacation time, she tended to go to exotic locations with her boyfriend and his friends, which made Samantha feel left out and neglected. She resented the time her mother spent with her boyfriend and was angry about her father's tendency toward violent behavior. In fact, Samantha felt as if she had no close attachments in her family.

Samantha was a gymnast, and being thin was necessary to her sport, but eating made her feel less lonely at home. She began eating in secret followed by forced vomiting, and this made her feel powerful—at least until her symptoms started to spiral out of control. No one noticed her bingeing and vomiting at home, but at school her friends started to take note of her tendency toward getting sick, especially after she "pigged out." One of her friends alerted the school guidance counselor, who helped get Samantha into treatment.

Samantha's therapist used an interpersonal approach, focusing on the interpersonal deficits inherent in her family of origin. At first, Samantha enjoyed the fuss her family made over her. Her mother spent less time with her boyfriend, and her father stopped being so angry all of the time. After a while, though, her parents' typical patterns returned, and the goal of individual therapy focused on analyzing these patterns, whereas the goal of family therapy focused on changing the patterns themselves. For example, Robyn and her mother had an enmeshed relationship, and Samantha felt caught in the middle of it. Therapy helped Samantha realize that the problems in their relationship were not her fault. Samantha's therapist also recommended individual therapy for Robyn and Samantha's father, but unfortunately neither of them followed through with the recommendation. However, they did become active participants in Samantha's treatment, and over the course of the next 2 years Samantha gained confidence in herself, was less preoccupied with her physical appearance, and completely stopped her purging behaviors.

Medication

Medication is not a first-line treatment for eating disorders, but it is used to treat the associated symptoms. For example, because depression frequently occurs in individuals with eating disorders, the use of antidepressants such as Prozac is often recommended. The research suggests that medication needs to be taken for a long period of time (at least 6 months) and that it should be used in conjunction with psychotherapy (i.e., CBT, family therapy, interpersonal therapy) and work with a nutritionist. Unfortunately, there is no drug that has

Common Techniques Used in Treatment

The following techniques are frequently used by therapists of different orientations in their treatment:

- food journaling in which patients are asked to keep a log of what, where, and when they eat as well as the thoughts and feelings they may have had;
- educating patients about food and eating habits by talking about the effect of purging on the body or the cultural factors that are involved in eating disorders;
- developing positive eating habits such as not skipping meals, eating with friends and family, and responding appropriately to the body's signs of hunger and fullness;
- setting realistic goals in terms of weight gain or decreasing bingeing and purging behaviors;
- improving body image by helping patients think differently about their bodies;
- identifying and challenging negative thoughts and feelings such as "I should be perfect" or "I'm a loser because I couldn't stop myself from eating the whole carton of ice cream"; and
- helping patients to establish healthy social relationships with their peers.

When Is Hospitalization Necessary?

Most patients with eating disorders are treated outside of the hospital setting, but your doctor may require hospitalization if your child

- is having a medical emergency (severe, quick weight loss or heart problems);
- cannot break a severe binge–starve cycle;
- needs to have a severe eating disorder evaluated more thoroughly and quickly than can typically be done on an outpatient basis, particularly if the child or family is in crisis; and
- has recently had, or threatened to have, a suicide attempt.

153

been shown to be effective at treating the actual symptoms of anorexia or bulimia, although psychiatric medications can have a useful place in the overall treatment approach because they address what is often an underlying depression and sometimes help give the client an increased ability to control her out-of-control eating behaviors.

CONCLUDING THOUGHTS

Eating disorders are serious conditions. If untreated, they can become chronic and pose serious problems to a child's health. These disorders tend to occur with other disorders, such as depression, anxiety, and obsessive–compulsive disorder, which can make them more difficult to treat. However, there are treatments that have been found to be effective, and having a multipronged approach that uses the skills of a psychologist, psychiatrist, primary care medical doctor, and nutritionist is of utmost importance. Psychological approaches often emphasize the importance of changes in family communication patterns, so it is important to enter treatment knowing that the entire family will likely play a part in the healing process. Finding an experienced team of professionals is one of the most important things that you can do. There are a number of resources in the appendix of this book that can be used as a beginning guide to understanding these disorders and possible treatment options. Your child's pediatrician or your family doctor is also a good resource for finding an experienced team of eating disorder professionals.

CHAPTER 10

OTHER PSYCHOLOGICAL PROBLEMS AND ISSUES

The reasons why parents might consult a psychologist to help with their children's problems are endless, and this chapter doesn't begin to cover the possibilities. However, the chapter does highlight various reasons parents might seek treatment. Some of these issues, such as psychosis, are quite serious, rare, and chronic, whereas others, such as peer relationship problems, are common and sometimes more situationally driven and transient. There any many instances in which parents consult a psychologist and there is no "diagnosis," yet psychological treatment and consultation can be quite helpful in dealing with life's ups and downs. Some children have difficulties adapting to school, the birth of a sibling, or the death of a loved one and behave in ways that are developmentally or situationally inappropriate. Parents don't always know which problems merit psychological attention and which ones are worthy of a wait-and-see approach. They may decide to consult with a professional to find out, and the "treatment" may consist of just a one-time consultation.

For example, Jerez was a 6-year-old boy with a history of eczema and picky eating. Jerez didn't just pick at his food, he had a habit of picking at his dry skin to the point that scabs formed and bled. His parents were not sure whether he was an odd child with unusual food patterns and a compulsive tendency to pick at his skin or whether his behaviors were within the normal range. They consulted with a psychologist who evaluated both of these irritating behaviors. The psychologist helped the parents identify what types of foods Jerez ate, and once they looked at their list they realized that although Jerez did not eat many things, he did eat enough things, and he ate foods from all of the major food groups—including vegetables. In terms of the picking habit, the psychologist told Jerez's parents that Jerez needed to take responsibility for his picking. In other words, he needed to carry band-aids in his pocket in case he picked his scabs until they bled. He needed to be responsible for keeping his skin clean and for putting ointment on his eczema. The psychologist gave them a number of tips and told them to call if things did not work out. The parents were surprised that these few suggestions—along with reassurance that his behavior was not abnormal—went a long way in helping Jerez. They did not need to see the psychologist again, although they knew that he would be available as needed.

What follows are snapshots of how psychological treatment can be useful for a number of different disorders. This is not an exhaustive list, nor does it provide all the answers you need if you suspect your child may have difficulties in one of these areas. However, if you want further information, consult the suggestions in Part III of this book. It offers a number of different resources to find answers to your questions.

SCHOOL PROBLEMS

Many children exhibit problems with school achievement. Many of these children have a learning disability or attention problem, but even children without learning or attentional problems can experience difficulties with school, particularly as these problems relate to poor study skills or organizational skills. For example, Francine had been a strong student until seventh grade, when she transferred from a public elementary school to a very competitive preparatory school. Her parents became quite concerned when in the middle of her seventh-grade year she did not receive any *A*s but instead received quite a few *C*s. Francine was struggling with organizing her studies and studying for tests. She was lacking the skills necessary for this difficult academic environment. Her parents consulted with an educational psychologist who evaluated her writing, study, and organizational skills and taught her ways to better structure her time and organize her notes. The educational psychologist worked closely with the school psychologist and educational resource center to provide Francine with continued support. Within a year Francine had learned the skills necessary to be a successful student. Although she did not have a diagnosable learning disability, she did display vulnerabilities in written language and study skills that necessitated treatment. It is possible that she may not have ever needed treatment had she not transferred to a competitive school environment; however, with the correct support she was found quite capable of success in completing challenging work.

FAMILY CONFLICT AND STRESSORS

Family relations are the earliest and most enduring relationships that children will have. They affect a child's competence, sense of well-being, and ability to adapt to changes in the environment. In the best situations, families provide children with positive benefits such as a supportive and nurturing environment that allows children to learn about secure attachments and gives them a positive sense of well-being. However, even the most supportive families have experiences and events that can be stressful, negative, and harmful to a child's development. Even the best parents can have difficulty coping with challenging children. We've all observed (or perhaps experienced!) the screaming child in the grocery store who is refusing to budge unless his mother buys him candy. Although most children will act this way at some point, for some children, this behavior is the norm. Coping with this type of child is not easy, and many parents rely on parenting methods from their own childhoods. Although these methods might be appropriate in some cases, in other cases they can involve inappropriate parenting methods such as verbal threats or physical coercion. Many of these parents can benefit from learning more appropriate parenting skills.

In addition, stressful events in the family affect different children in different ways. For example, when Carrie's parents went through a painful divorce, she became a more responsible 12-year-old. Her 13-year-old brother, Chase, had the opposite reaction in that he started to misbehave and exhibit conduct problems. Chase's mother sought more intensive treatment for Chase but only consulted a few times with a therapist for Carrie. Certain situations tend to trigger more intense reactions than others. Living in an abusive household can be much more stressful than being bullied at school, yet children in both of these situations may benefit from treatment. Similarly, problems such as a chronic illness in a parent or sibling, a move to a new school, or a death of a loved one may require treatment, although most of the time children adapt to these situations without psychological support.

Overall, treatment of stress and family conflict tends to provide parents with assistance in one or more of the following areas:

- providing parents with a better knowledge of their child's development and what they can expect from their children based on their age and developmental level;
- helping parents develop ways to cope with stress, particularly as it relates to parenting young children;

- assisting parents in learning better communication patterns;
- providing parents with knowledge about home management;
- helping parents negotiate parenting duties;
- putting parents in contact with appropriate social, educational, and health services as needed; and
- teaching parents the most appropriate and effective discipline techniques.

PEER RELATIONSHIP PROBLEMS

Friendships and peer groups are important aspects of children's development. Most of us have struggled at some point with issues such as popularity and peer acceptance, and sometimes these struggles can leave children feeling depressed, rejected, and confused. For example, Molly was a popular girl until fifth grade when her "best" friend, Cindy, started ignoring her. Molly's other friends soon followed Cindy's lead, and Molly found herself sitting alone at the lunch table and playing by herself on the playground. When Molly and her mother arrived in my office, Molly's mother explained that Molly was crying herself to sleep at night and did not want to go to school in the morning. Treatment with Molly involved not only talking with Molly but also working with the teacher and school guidance counselor to develop a plan to help the girls in Molly's class manage these issues.

In contrast, Thomas's mom came to my office worried because Thomas, a seventh grader, was acting like a bully. She was worried that he was "too popular" and that he could "get away with doing anything to anyone." The school guidance counselor had contacted her because Thomas was being perceived as a bully, and although it seemed as if Thomas had many friends, most of these "friends" were just afraid of him. The guidance counselor worked weekly with Thomas to help him find ways of socializing with his peers without resorting to fear tactics. In the course of therapy, it was found that

Thomas was actually not feeling so good about himself. In fact, Thomas had difficulty with many aspects of school, particularly reading and writing, and Thomas's bullying behaviors were his attempts to feel more powerful because he was feeling weak academically. Treatment for Thomas included providing him with tutoring in reading and writing to help him feel more confident in the school environment.

OBESITY

Obesity is an important health problem, and rates of childhood obesity have increased considerably over the past 30 years. Obesity is associated with many physical problems, such as diabetes and heart disease, and social and psychological difficulties, including behavior problems and depression. Children who are perceived as overweight are less liked than their thinner peers, and they are sometimes described as "lazy" or "stupid." In addition, children who are obese tend not to participate in physical activities, such as team sports, and this lack of participation can make them feel even more socially isolated. These types of experiences can affect self-esteem.

   Although many obese children do not have adjustment difficulties or problems with self-esteem, some do, and most obese children could benefit from some assistance in helping them change their behaviors. These issues are rarely just the child's problem because family, dietary, and social factors are often important in the development of obesity. Children observe and imitate the behaviors of the adults around them. For example, Bobby was a 9-year-old who was 60% overweight for his height and age. His pediatrician referred him to a weight control treatment program. Bobby's problems with weight were chronic and becoming worse. Bobby's parents were quite concerned, and his father felt guilty because he too was overweight and had struggled with these issues from a young age. Treatment at the weight clinic included family meetings at which family members learned about food intake and exercise and began to keep a food journal. What they found was alarming; Bobby snacked frequently on high-calorie snack foods, particularly after school while his parents were still at work. The family also had to come to terms with the fact that sometimes they "sabotaged" Bobby's efforts to lose weight; family activities often revolved around high-calorie foods, and Bobby's mother frequently cooked his favorite deserts as a way to cheer him up. Therapy included changing not only Bobby's eating habits but also the family's lifestyle choices. It provided his parents with the skills necessary to help Bobby maintain his weight loss once he had met his treatment goals. As an added benefit to Bobby's successful treatment, Bobby's father lost weight as well.

ELIMINATION DISORDERS

The term *elimination disorders* is a fancy way of saying toilet training problems. It is common for children to exhibit some difficulties in becoming toilet trained, and although parents solve many of these difficulties on their own, professional assistance is sometimes sought when these difficulties become serious enough. The usual sequence of toilet training is nighttime bowel control, daytime bowel control, daytime bladder control, and, finally, nighttime bladder control. Children typically complete this sequence by the age of 36 months, but some children display problems with daytime and/or nighttime wetting (known as *enuresis*) far after this age. Other children may pass feces into their clothing or other unacceptable places. After the age of 4 years, this is referred to as *encopresis*.

For instance, Sally was an exuberant 10-year-old who, since the age of 3½ years, never had a toileting accident during the day.

161

However, she wet her bed 4 or 5 nights of the week. She did not have any medical or psychological issues that would explain her problems in this area, although her dad did wet the bed until he was 12 years old. As Sally grew, her problems with bedwetting were getting in the way of her social relationships in that she was embarrassed to spend the night at a friend's house. After a thorough checkup at her pediatrician's office, her pediatrician prescribed a urine alarm system whereby an alarm sounds when the child begins to void. The alarm wakes the child (and parents) up, and the child is taught to turn off the alarm and to go to the bathroom to finish urinating. This simple treatment has been found to be quite effective.

Roger was a 6-year-old who had been soiling his pants nearly every day since he was a baby. After a very careful medical evaluation, it was determined that Roger was quite constipated (as most children with encopresis are) and that he had learned to retain feces because he had experienced anxiety and pain with toileting in the past, only to void at inappropriate times. This was a source of considerable anxiety and distress for Roger and his parents. When Roger and his parents came to the psychologist's office for an initial evaluation, Roger went into an empty office (while his parents were talking to the psychologist) and had a bowel movement under the desk. As should be evident, Roger's problems were not just in the toileting realm, and many children with encopresis have other psychological and behavior problems as well. Roger's treatment included both medical (i.e., increasing fiber, taking laxatives) and behavior management (i.e., scheduling regular toilet times). Treatment can also include therapy for the child with encopresis and parent guidance sessions. Positive consequences were provided as rewards when Roger used the toilet appropriately. As is true for many children with encopresis, Roger's behavior problems improved after he was able to manage his toileting in an age-appropriate manner.

SLEEP DISORDERS

There are many types of sleep disorders that are of concern to psychologists who work with children. Most of these involve difficulty getting to sleep and staying asleep. Less commonly, a psychologist might be asked to treat problems with sleepwalking, sleep terrors, or nightmares. A number of different treatments have been found to be effective in treating sleep problems. For children who have trouble getting to sleep, their parents are taught to establish bedtime routines that encourage a child to fall asleep. In cases of sleep terrors and sleepwalking, treatment usually is not indicated because the episodes usually stop as suddenly as they start. However, parents frequently consult their pediatricians and psychologists for education and support. With regard to nightmares, treatments that target anxiety reduction have been found to be effective because nightmares are frequently a reaction to anxiety-provoking events.

SUBSTANCE USE

Substance use, which includes the use of alcohol, tobacco, and illegal drugs, is a very serious problem that is far beyond the scope of this book. Substance use can be part of larger behavior problems,

Sleep Terrors

Sleep terrors are common in about 3% of children ages 4 to 12 years. Sleep terrors occur when a child is in deep sleep, which is usually around 2 hours after falling asleep. During the sleep terror, the child sits upright in bed and starts screaming. Although the child looks quite distressed, the child most often does not fully awaken and usually has no memory of the event. These are in contrast to nightmares, which are frightening dreams common in children from ages 3 to 6 years and which the child typically does remember.

such as antisocial behavior or conduct disorder. However, the use of substances such as alcohol, tobacco, and marijuana is common among adolescents who do not have other problems because many adolescents experiment with substance use. This presents a challenge for parents and psychologists in that it can be difficult to determine whether a child is engaging in experimentation that may be developmentally normative or in patterns that have much more serious consequences. Studies of adolescent behaviors have shown that over half of adolescents have tried an illicit drug by the time they finish high school, and most adolescents experiment with more than one substance. Over one third have done so by the end of eighth grade. Marijuana is the most widely used illicit drug, but about 20% of high school seniors will have tried a drug other than marijuana at some point during high school. Statistics regarding adolescent substance abuse are also concerning because 62% of 12th graders and 21% of eighth graders report being drunk at least once in their life. In addition, about 25% of 12th graders are cigarette smokers.

Treatment approaches vary depending on the type of substance used and the frequency of the use. Sometimes parents will seek the services of a psychologist because they found their 14-year-old smoking pot in the basement with her friends. Although the child "swears" that it is the first time, the parents are alarmed enough to seek professional help. Depending on the circumstances, long-term treatment may not be indicated or the psychologist may assess the situation and find that the child's behavior is a symptom of a more serious issue that needs intensive treatment. Treatment of these issues is best left to professionals who specialize in treating alcohol and drug use. Most treatment programs address multiple influences, such as peer relationships, family functioning, schools, neighborhood, and community. The stakes can be high when dealing with these issues, and the problems can be hard to treat; thus, spending the time to find the right specialist (or specialist team) is important.

PSYCHOSIS

Of all the possible problems mentioned in this chapter, this one is the most serious. Fortunately it is quite rare. Psychotic disorders are sometimes referred to as *thought disorders,* and their defining characteristic is significant problems in the ability to perceive and respond appropriately to reality. Children with thought disorders, or psychosis, may report seeing things that are not there (also referred to as *visual hallucinations*), smelling things that are not there (*olfactory hallucinations*), hearing things that are not there (*auditory hallucinations*), and/or feeling things that are not there (*tactile hallucinations*). In fact, children and adults are not typically diagnosed with a psychotic disorder unless they experience some type of hallucination. As you might guess, children and adolescents who experience a thought disorder generally are displaying significant problems in *reality testing,* or the ability to discern what is real from what is imagined.

Children who are experiencing a thought disorder will usually display problems in their ability to communicate with others. Their speech may be *pressured* in that they speak rapidly. Their thoughts may be *tangential*—off topic or irrelevant to the conversation. They may move rapidly from one topic to another, and their thoughts may seem illogical. Symptoms can also include paranoia, odd behaviors, excessive concerns about their body, and very disorganized behaviors. Other symptoms that parents may observe include social withdrawal, sleep disturbances, suicidal thoughts, and problems with attention. Sometimes this constellation of symptoms indicates a child is showing early signs of schizophrenia. Other times, these symptoms occur when a child is exhibiting significant symptoms of depression and anxiety.

Sabina was a 14-year-old girl who had experienced significant symptoms of anxiety and obsessive–compulsive disorder from age 7. Her symptoms were well controlled with medication and psychotherapy. However, when she started high school, she began to experience very severe anxiety to the point that she thought she heard voices telling her she was "bad, stupid, and ugly." She felt her math teacher was laughing at her every time he turned around to write on the chalkboard. Sabina knew these thoughts were "crazy," but she could not do anything to stop them. Sabina's psychiatrist changed her medications to medications that treated her current symptoms. Soon thereafter, she reported feeling no psychotic symptoms.

In contrast, Lee was a 15-year-old boy whose grandfather had schizophrenia. Lee began behaving in strange ways; he refused to shower, and his parents found him talking to the bedroom wall at random times. He refused to see his friends and spent most of his free time in the basement. His grades plummeted, and he began skipping school. Despite the fact that Lee's grandfather had schizophrenia (and schizophrenia can be genetically transmitted), Lee's parents hoped that this was just "typical adolescent angst." It was not until Lee attempted to jump in front of a moving train (because he was "told to do it by the voices in his head") that he was hospitalized and diagnosed with a thought disorder that was likely an early sign of schizophrenia.

Thought disorders can be the sign of a lifelong mental health disability (as is quite possible for Lee), or they can be a transient problem (as in Sabina's case). In either case, psychotic symptoms can appear or become exacerbated during stressful times of life. It is difficult to predict anyone's ultimate outcome. Treatment usually consists of a combination of medication, therapy, and life skills training. It typically involves the services of a medical doctor (usually a child psychiatrist) and a mental health professional (e.g., child psychologist). If parents suspect that their child may be exhibiting problems with thinking, immediate consultation with a doctor is advised because these problems may also be indications of medical problems such as a brain tumor or stroke.

CONCLUDING THOUGHTS

Childhood and adolescence are filled with extreme behaviors. In fact, most of us who look back on our childhood can remember feeling extreme emotions and behaving in ways that were out of character. However, sometimes parents become concerned when they feel their children are developing in ways that are less than optimal. This chapter provided a "flavor" of the types of issues that might lead a parent to a psychologist's office. There is a fine line between what is considered normal versus problematic. However, it is never a bad idea to get consultation if you are worried that your child might be displaying behaviors that make you feel a need for help. Sometimes one appointment can set your mind at ease. At other times consulting with a psychologist can lead to longer term, but necessary, treatment. In either case, the expertise of a qualified professional can help you determine what is best for your child and provide your child with the important tools for more successful development.

Part III

THE TREATMENTS

CHAPTER 11

PSYCHOTHERAPY: INTERPERSONAL AND INSIGHT-ORIENTED APPROACHES

When you think of therapy, do you think of someone lying on a couch with a bearded doctor sitting behind taking notes and saying, "hmm" and "tell me more about that?" Many people do, but that type of therapy, known as *psychoanalysis,* is actually rarely used with children and represents only one of the types of therapy used with adults. However, the therapies explored in this chapter come closest to that idea because they are generally *insight oriented* in that the goal is for patients to gain insight into their difficulties and for this insight to lead to changes in the problematic behaviors. Three different approaches are explained in the chapter: interpersonal therapy (IPT), psychodynamic psychotherapy, and play therapy.

INTERPERSONAL THERAPY

IPT was originally developed to treat adult depression but has since been used to treat children and adolescents. Its underlying idea is that the quality of a person's relationships can cause, maintain, or provide a shield against life's stressors and help the child cope more effectively with a range of psychological symptoms and issues. The main goals of IPT are to decrease the child's problematic symptoms and improve the quality of his or her significant relationships. During the course of therapy, the psychologist will help the child or adolescent identify the main *problem area* (see the next paragraph). Once the problem area is defined, the therapist will help identify effective communication skills and techniques that help the child cope with and manage the problem area. Once these techniques are identified, the child will practice these during the session and (eventually) outside the session, use these skills in his relationships.

IPT defines problem areas as falling into one or more of four possible areas: *grief* (severe mourning or sorrow from a loss), *interpersonal role disputes* (e.g., the type of fights that occur between parents and adolescent children), *role transitions* (e.g., the transition from childhood to adolescence), and *interpersonal deficits* (difficulty relating to other children that can lead to chronic isolation). The child or adolescent will learn over the course of therapy not only which problem area(s) affects her, but also how these affect her. For example, depressed adolescents don't typically handle social roles well, and that makes matters more complicated for them. For instance, Nancy was a 16-year-old whose serious depression caused her to be irritable with her teachers and socially isolated from her peers. Thus, treatment needed to focus on how to get along better with her teachers and how to become more socially engaged with her peers.

What Is the Typical Course of Therapy?

IPT is a brief time-limited therapy that has three phases. In Phase 1, which typically takes the first two or three sessions, the therapist establishes a framework for treatment and educates the patient about his or her difficulties. For example, the patient might learn that depression is not due to laziness or "not trying hard enough to pull yourself up by your bootstraps" (as one patient's father said) but an illness that sometimes has a medical basis. During this first phase of treatment, the patient and therapist make a contract for a specific number of sessions, and the treatment focuses on the here and now. This is quite different from the other treatments that are explained later in this chapter.

The sessions of Phase 2 revolve around the treatment itself. The focus of treatment depends on how the problem area is defined. For example, if grief is the issue, the therapist will facilitate mourning. Teddy was a 12-year-old whose mother died a year before he came to therapy, and this event (along with unresolved grief) was thought to be the reason for his depression. The therapy consisted of helping Teddy mourn his mother's passing by talking about the event and his memories (both positive and negative) of her. If the problem is defined as stemming from a role dispute, therapy may consist of determining the nature of the dispute and finding ways to resolve it. For example, parents and adolescents may have differing opinions about what constitutes appropriate behavior and could benefit from resolving these issues. If the problem is defined as a role transition, the child may need to learn and evaluate the positive and negative aspects of the change. For example, an adolescent who is having trouble leaving home to go to college may benefit from talking through the positive and negative things he is experiencing or expecting to experience. Finally, if the problem falls in the interpersonal deficit domain, therapy may focus on defining the problematic social skills and helping the child develop appropriate social skills.

As you might have guessed, treatment often focuses on more than one of these areas. For example, Teddy's therapy focused primarily on helping him process unresolved grief even though he and his father also had difficulty with role disputes because his father thought that Teddy should be "pulling his own weight" around the house. Some of Teddy's father's expectations were unrealistic, and others were not, and the therapist helped Teddy and his father identify which were appropriate.

Phase 3 of IPT focuses on reviewing the child's achievements and acknowledging the gains he has made. The therapist also helps define what to watch out for—what symptoms might be a warning sign of a recurrence of symptoms. Some time is spent talking about how to generalize the skills learned to future situations. Interestingly enough, if the patient has not improved by the end of therapy, IPT views the "failure" as a problem with the treatment, not with the patient, and the therapist would discuss other treatment options, which could include cognitive behavior therapy (CBT) or medication (among other options).

What Disorders Are Effectively Treated With Interpersonal Therapy?

IPT is used to treat a variety of disorders, but it has been shown to be most effective in treating depression. A number of studies have demonstrated the efficacy of IPT for adult depression. For example, a study of 250 depressed adults compared IPT with CBT, medication, and a placebo. CBT and IPT were found to be equally effective for treating depression but were not quite as effective as medication. In a study that evaluated adults with more severe depression, however, IPT was found to be more effective than CBT. Fewer studies have been completed with adolescents (and virtually none with children), but those that have been completed have demonstrated that adolescents

> Who is qualified to do these types of therapies? Insight-oriented therapies are performed not only by psychologists but also by psychiatrists, psychiatric social workers, licensed professional counselors, and psychiatric nurses who should have specialized training in one of these methods.

treated with IPT have been found to have a decrease in depressive symptoms, improved social functioning, and better peer relationships. Among severely depressed teens, the data were quite similar to those found in adults; the adolescents in the IPT group did significantly better than adolescents who received supportive therapy. Some studies have shown that combining IPT with medication yields even better results in adults with mood disorders, and current studies are underway to evaluate this possibility in adolescent populations. Overall, IPT is a therapy that teaches patients how to cope with their problems and thus might reduce the risk of relapse.

PSYCHODYNAMIC PSYCHOTHERAPY

In psychodynamic psychotherapy, the goal is to achieve insight into the patient's problems by bringing unconscious, confusing, or unclear information into his or her awareness. In comparison with psychoanalytic psychotherapy (see the exhibit that follows), much more attention is given to the realities of current life than to dreams and the unconscious, although dreams and unconscious thoughts are explored. Interpretation is an important component of this treatment. For example, the psychologist might make an interpretation by articulating the coping strategy that the child is currently using, which may not be a positive way of coping at all. In addition, a central feature of this treatment is the child's relationship with the therapist. Through a caring, trusting relationship, the child will feel comfortable expressing his wishes, fears, and conflicts. This allows the therapist to interpret the child's thoughts, feelings, and behaviors. In younger children, play is used as a way to uncover these feelings and conflicts (for more information, see the section titled Play Therapy); whereas in older children, talking to the therapist is the primary mode of treatment.

What Is Psychoanalysis?

Psychoanalysis is a type of therapy in which the patient usually reclines on a couch, and the therapist (analyst) sits behind the patient so that nonverbal cues and eye contact cannot influence the patient's *free associations*. Free association is the primary process of the therapy. The patient is instructed to freely say whatever comes to mind, whether it be dreams, fantasies, memories, wishes, thoughts, or feelings (even positive or negative feelings about the therapist). The analyst typically has a neutral, quiet, and non-judgmental stance, and the aim of therapy is to uncover as much as possible about how the patient's mind works. This therapy usually requires three to five meetings a week and requires a commitment of at least 2 to 3 years. It has not been empirically proved to be effective in treating problems in children and adolescents. Thus, the cost (both in time and money) of this treatment is not usually justified for the treatment of childhood behavior problems and disorders. That being said, there are some gifted child psychoanalysts who are quite successful in treating children. The success of their treatment may have more to do with the positive qualities of the therapist than the mode of treatment.

What Is the Typical Course of Therapy?

Psychodynamic therapy with children and adolescents typically begins with an interview with the parents, followed by a diagnostic evaluation (often an interview) with the child. When the child is still young enough to play with toys, the form of the interview might be through playing with the child and observing the child's choice of play materials and the nature of her play. It is thought that the child projects her personality and conflicts on to the materials in a meaningful way.

Olivia was an 8-year-old girl who had complained of headaches since her father was killed by a drunk driver a year ago. She had completed a battery of medical tests that indicated no medical cause for her headaches. Her pediatrician referred her to a psycho-dynamically trained psychologist to help determine possible reasons for her difficulties. When Olivia arrived with her mother for her first meeting, she refused to answer any questions about her dad. When she walked into the playroom, she immediately started playing with the toy cars, crashing one into another and saying, "These cars are bad, they need to be killed." Over the course of therapy, which lasted 2 years, the therapist would help Olivia to understand her feelings of anger, their origin, and the conflict she had about these feelings, which contributed to the development of her headaches. Week after week, Olivia would arrive and play out her aggression toward cars and "bad people." She sometimes would get mad at her therapist for not "keeping the bad people out of the cars." Over time, though, her play became less focused on this theme, and she began to talk about her feelings more directly. The therapist provided a warm, safe, and comfortable environment, validated and understood her feelings, and over time helped her express these feelings verbally and appropriately. This led to the resolution of her headaches as well as working through the feelings of anger, grief, and loss surrounding the death of her dad.

What Disorders Are Effectively Treated With Psychodynamic Psychotherapy?

Unfortunately, there is little empirical evidence that shows that psychodynamic psychotherapy works in treating childhood disorders. This does not mean that it does not work, only that there is little research-based proof that it does. There have been a few recent studies indicating that short-term psychodynamic psychotherapy is helpful in treating depression in children (when compared with children in a control group). More research is needed, however, and there are some drawbacks to this approach. First, it can be a time consuming and costly process. Second, psychologists do not know which disorders can be effectively treated with this approach. Third, this type of therapy can really only be used with children and adolescents who are verbal and can express themselves through language. Thus, it's not particularly useful for children who have language or cognitive deficits.

Nevertheless, many children and families believe that this type of therapy made a huge positive difference in their lives. What can account for this positive change? Research has shown that regardless of the type of therapy, the establishment of a special relationship between therapist and patient is vital to positive change, along with the effort that the therapist makes in bringing about positive changes in the child's feelings, behaviors, and thoughts. Thus, it may be that the special quality of the relationship is what makes the difference in the outcome of many treatments. Furthermore, just because a psychologist specializes in psychodynamic psychotherapy does not mean that is the only treatment he or she uses. For example, a psychodynamic psychotherapist may use cognitive behavior techniques to help a child cope with symptoms of anxiety, and this type of approach can be quite effective. Many child therapists are quite open, or *eclectic,* in their treatment and even though they subscribe to one major point of view, will incorporate other perspectives according to of the needs of the child.

PLAY THERAPY

There are many different forms of (and schools of thought regarding) play therapy, but all types of play therapy use toys, puppets, dolls, blocks, Legos, Play-Doh, and games to help the child identify, talk about, and work through his feelings. Although it can be used as a stand-alone treatment, psychologists of many orientations may use play at different points in the therapy process to help them better identify, understand, and manage a child's conflicts, feelings, and behaviors. Play therapy is typically used with children from the ages of 3 to 11 years. Sometimes play therapy takes place in a fully equipped playroom, although that setting isn't essential. What is necessary is that the child has ready access to play materials that encourage the expression of his or her needs, feelings, and experiences. Throughout the play process, the therapist will help the child explore difficult real-life experiences (with or without the child's verbalization), express and explore a wide range of feelings, and experience successful outcomes and resolutions in his or her play.

Play therapy is not an "anything goes" approach because children do not feel safe in a relationship with no boundaries. Although a certain amount of messiness is accepted, a child is not allowed to break the crayons or spill paint all over the room. The therapist might say to the child at that point,

> It looks like you would like to break all those crayons, but that is not what the crayons are for. Drawing is what crayons are for. Maybe you could draw a picture for me of how it would feel to break those crayons so we can better understand your feelings.

Through this type of interchange, the therapist recognizes the child's frustration while suggesting an alternative to the behavior and also asserting the boundaries of the relationship.

What Is the Typical Course of Therapy?

A play therapist will typically begin by taking a complete history of the child from the parents. During the first session, the therapist will describe what to expect in treatment, how the parent will be involved in the treatment (parenting sessions) and how much the treatment will cost. Once the therapist feels she understands the problem (through the parents' eyes) and how if affects the child and family, the actually therapy process will begin. Most play therapists see their patients one to two times a week (sometimes more). The actual length of treatment varies depending on the child and the severity of his or her problems. Therapy usually ends when the child's level of functioning returns to normal.

What Disorders Are Effectively Treated by Play Therapy?

There is not much empirical data validating play therapy as a particularly effective approach in treating most childhood behavior and emotional problems. However, it has been successfully used by insight-oriented child therapists and is also frequently used for children who have experienced trauma and who have difficulty talking about their experiences (but who may be able to "enact" their experiences).

Joey was an 8-year-old who had suffered burns over 70% of his body during a house fire. He had been in the hospital for 4 months but never once discussed anything about the accident or the future. His psychologist used nondirective play therapy techniques as a way of helping him talk about his feelings. Joey would frequently gravitate toward playing with the army men who would fight the bad guys. Sometimes the good guys would "catch on fire" and need to be rescued by the doctors. Session after session, Joey would reenact these scenes until one day he said to his psychologist, "You know, I was in a fire too," and at that point he was ready to talk about his feelings and about some of the things that had frightened him and were worrying him about the future.

Studies have demonstrated that play therapy has been helpful for children whose parents are divorcing, and for children with attention-deficit/hyperactivity disorder. In both of these studies, the therapy was short term (fewer than 20 sessions) and quite directive. For example, in the study on children with attention-deficit/hyperactivity disorder, the researchers used a particular game (Self-Control Game) to increase the children's self-perception of their self-control. Although play therapy can be useful for some children, it is not the treatment of first choice for most problem areas. If your child has an anxiety disorder or phobia, play therapy might actually be counterproductive because the child may spend months (even years) in play therapy trying to "process" his problems, whereas a 10-week course of CBT (see Chapter 13, this volume) would likely have been successful.

How Do I Find a Good Therapist?

The best way to find a good therapist is to ask people you trust for their recommendations—but that's only a starting point. Some psychologists will meet with you for a free complementary session before you commit to entering treatment. You might want to meet with a few before you commit or at least talk with them by phone to interview them about their training, experience, and treatment approach. Unfortunately, child psychologists are in great demand, and you might find yourself waiting longer than you'd like for an appointment. Don't let that discourage you or stop you from searching for the best person. You might be working with this person for a long time, and it's better to wait to find the right person for you and your child than to go to the first available person.

If you have met with one or more psychologists for an initial visit, your next step is to choose the one you are most comfortable with and try out a few visits. Be honest with the therapist if you are not ready to commit. In other words, tell him, "I'm not sure this is the route I want to go, but I'd like to try two or three sessions to figure out if it is." If after the first three sessions, you don't have a good feeling, it's probably better to move on to someone else. Finding a therapist who will work with both you and your child is essential to a successful treatment outcome. You should feel like part of the therapy team and feel supported and cared for. You should also feel that the therapist has much to offer in terms of insight into your child's problems, a plan for how he is going to help treat those problems, and coping skills for you and your child that will help you deal with the issues on a daily basis.

The Therapy Does Not Seem to Be Working. Should I Try Something New?

This question is a complicated one because in child therapy both the child and the child's parents need to be comfortable with the therapist. So it's possible for you to think the psychologist is wonderful but for your child to think the reverse. In addition, the therapist will sometimes bring up issues that are difficult for you to hear, and you might find yourself angry at or disliking the therapist. At other times, you might find yourself jealous of the relationship your child has with the therapist. These feelings are completely normal, but often when you are questioning the treatment, your instincts are telling you that something isn't working. My best advice is for you to trust your instincts but make sure your own issues (e.g., feelings of jealously) are not coloring your instincts. If you are finding that more often than not you are questioning whether the treatment is working, it probably is not.

The best thing to do when you feel like this is to discuss your thoughts with the therapist. The therapist may actually have a very good answer as to why she thinks the treatment has hit a standstill. On the other hand, the therapist might say, "I'm also worried that the treatment isn't working and I, too, have been concerned as to what to do." It is a bad sign if you find the therapist is defensive. Even if the therapist thinks you are wrong (i.e., thinks the treatment is going along fine), he should not challenge your feelings of concern. You know your child best, and you should not feel you need to stick with a therapist when your gut is telling you the therapy is not working for your child. If you cannot find a resolution to this issue, it is probably an indication to move on. I have seen too many parents who have tearfully told me, "I knew we weren't getting anywhere with Dr. X, but he kept telling me to be patient, and now Johnny is more depressed than ever." If your child is anxious, has been in therapy for a year, and is as anxious as ever, it is time to move on and seek a second opinion.

CONCLUDING THOUGHTS

Insight-oriented therapies have been used for many years to treat a host of different problems in children and adults. These therapies help the child gain insight into his or her difficulties, and it is hoped that this insight will lead to changes in the difficult behaviors. The research on these therapies in children is not as comprehensive as the research on other therapies, but insight-oriented therapies can still be quite helpful for a number of problems. It is important to make sure you see positive changes in your child's problematic behavior after he or she has been in treatment, although the changes may take months to observe. It is also important to remember that regardless of the therapy (whether this therapy or others that follow in Chapters 12–15, this volume), the special relationship between the therapist and the patient is vital to positive outcomes. Thus, make sure you feel comfortable and confident with not only the therapeutic approach but also the therapist. With the right treatment and the right person, major changes can occur, and these changes can be life changing for your child and your family.

CHAPTER 12

COGNITIVE BEHAVIOR THERAPY

Jack was a 15-year-old high school sophomore who had been experiencing depression for 6 months. His pediatrician referred him to a psychiatrist who prescribed Prozac for his depressive symptoms. However, his psychiatrist also thought he might benefit from the addition of cognitive behavior therapy (CBT) because of the research that has demonstrated that cognitive therapy combined with medication is more effective than either alone.

When Jack first arrived in his psychologist's office, he was irritable, thought "life isn't worth living," had stopped doing things he used to enjoy, and had negative thoughts about himself and his life. Jack was much harder on himself than he was on other people. When asked about friends, he answered, "I don't have any because I just don't fit in with those geeks." When asked about what kinds of plans he had after college, he replied, "High school sucks, and college will probably be worse. What's the use?"

Jack's pediatrician recommended a CBT approach because it is one that has been found to be effective for a number of disorders in children and is quite effective in treating depression. CBT views psychological problems as stemming from problems with faulty thought patterns, learning, and environmental experiences. The underlying premise is that the way children and adolescents think about their environment determines how they will react to it. The major goals of CBT are to identify maladaptive thoughts (or *cognitions*) and replace them with more adaptive ones, to teach children to use better coping strategies, and to help children be aware of and regulate their own behavior. Using a cognitive behavioral approach, Jack's therapist would help him learn to think more positively and use more effective social skills and coping strategies.

CBT is a highly collaborative therapy whereby the child and therapist together try to understand the problems the child is having and make a plan for addressing the problems. This therapy is not just about talking about problems—it is about doing something about them. As indicated previously, a core principle is that what people think about themselves impacts how they feel about themselves and their situation. CBT provides a way for children to closely examine and change the interpretations of their experiences that are faulty and that are causing them problems. It is not just about positive thinking but also about a way of *rethinking*.

It is helpful to see how this plays out in Jack's case. The beginning of therapy focused on assessing Jack's difficulties. Although the therapy focused on Jack, the therapist also spent time talking with Jack's parents. During the assessment phase of therapy, the therapist wanted to find out *what* the problem behaviors were, *when* they occurred, *where* they occurred, and *how often* they occurred. In Jack's case, the problem behavior was primarily depressed mood, and it was occurring most of the time, but the problems were most acutely felt when he was in school. Jack's therapist had him keep a record of the thoughts he was having, along with the behaviors and feelings that were present. Jack was happy to record this on his iPhone. Once Jack was able to record the situations, thoughts, and feelings that went along with his moodiness, he was able to look for patterns in his thinking. For example, Jack attended a private school, but he saw himself as a more "independent-thinking, artistic" student who did not fit into the "preppy, perfect-student" environment. Instead of embracing that difference, he developed the idea that he was "less than" the other students and called himself a "loser." He began to isolate himself and was not involved in any extra-curricular activities. Because of this, he had no opportunities to build new connections with other adolescents like himself, which might have led him to challenge his own beliefs about himself. The fact that "no one called [him] to hang out" only reinforced his belief that he was a loser.

Jack was able to break this cycle of isolation and self-loathing because his therapist helped him recognize and correct the errors in his thinking. This is a process called *cognitive restructuring*—in other words, Jack learned to rebuild the ways he was thinking about himself and his environment. Some of this was done within the 1-hour per week therapy session, and some was done through homework assignments. Homework is an important component of CBT because the therapy assumes that what happens between the sessions is just as important as what happens within them. During the session, the therapist would challenge Jack's beliefs. For example, when Jack said something like, "I'm a complete failure," or "No one loves me," the therapist would look at whether that was true or false by looking at the evidence for it. Some of these were clearly false, whereas others, such as "My math teacher doesn't like me," were somewhat true, and it was helpful for Jack to see the difference between the two. In addition, the therapist also asked Jack to start making a daily schedule so that he would start to get out of the house. Over time, his depressive symptoms started to lessen as his therapist helped him observe each positive day or experience as building blocks that energized him toward his goals.

CBT has been shown to be quite effective for children and adolescents who have a number of different disorders. What is common to the treatment strategy for all of these disorders is that the children and adolescents are made aware of the distorted perceptions and logic that cause them to have inaccurate or unrealistic views of the world around them. The therapist then works to challenge their faulty beliefs by teaching them, modeling different thoughts and approaches, and giving the child a chance to practice new thoughts and responses during therapy and in real-life situations. Cognitive therapy can be used alone, typically by a therapist who has specific training in CBT, or along with other therapies as part of a broader treatment plan. However, there are differences in the way the therapy is applied to different disorders.

COGNITIVE BEHAVIOR THERAPY FOR ANXIETY DISORDER

Linda was a 10th-grade student who constantly complained that she had trouble sleeping at night. She was an exceptionally strong student, but she tended to stay up writing and rewriting her homework and her class notes. Once she finally went to bed (sometimes as late as 2 a.m.), she had trouble "shutting [her] mind down." Although she was only in 10th grade, she had already started to worry about the college admission process. The worry caused her to have migraines and backaches. When she began having difficulties concentrating, she started to worry that her schoolwork was going to suffer. Her mother was also concerned, and she contacted Linda's pediatrician, who referred her to a cognitive behavior therapist.

Cognitive therapy for anxiety has been found to be quite effective. Linda's treatment focused on a number of different areas.

- Linda's therapist used cognitive restructuring, which helped Linda look at her schoolwork and future college applications as less threatening and which made her more likely to actually do the applications as opposed to worrying about doing them.

- Training in *relaxation and imagery* was an important component of treatment. During this component of treatment, Linda learned how to recognize the early signals of anxiety and then use relaxation methods to stop the cycle.
- Linda and her therapist discussed more adaptive ways of coping with her schoolwork. For example, did she need to recopy her notes? Was it vital that she hand in the perfect paper every time? What would happen if she received a B+ or A− once in a while?

Linda made very good progress with CBT, and although she initially refused medication, after a few weeks without making much progress, she decided to try a medication to make her "feel less uptight." Within several weeks of starting Luvox, Linda was feeling calmer and more confident. She found the therapy effective and within 3 months was falling asleep with little difficulty, reporting few headaches, and was much less anxious about her grades.

COGNITIVE BEHAVIOR THERAPY FOR DEPRESSION

Marty was a 9-year-old boy who was feeling sad more days than most. Although he had been an avid participant in karate and enthusiastically played the piano, over the past 4 months he had lost interest in both of these pursuits. Most days he had difficulty getting out of bed; his mother said, "He'd sleep all day if I'd let him." Marty's teacher noticed a significant drop in his school performance and called his mother to find out what was wrong. As it turned out, Marty had been feeling depressed ever since his father left the family and moved to a different state 6 months before. Marty's mother admitted that she too had been quite depressed and felt guilty that she had not noticed Marty's difficulties. It is fortunate that she found a therapist who was trained in therapeutic techniques that have been found to be effective in treating depression in children and adolescents.

CBT is widely recognized as being a successful treatment for mild to moderate depression. When applied to depression, CBT aims to challenge maladaptive beliefs and to enhance problem-solving and social skills. Marty's treatment focused on the following areas:

- recognizing and changing his irrational thoughts (e.g., Marty felt that if he had only been "a better son," his dad would not have left; his therapist helped him see how irrational this idea was),
- adopting more appropriate or positive responses to his own and to others' thoughts and feelings,
- improving his social and problem-solving skills (e.g., Marty focused on how best to cope with his schoolwork and what he could do when he started to feel socially isolated), and
- planning appropriate social activities and reengaging in extra-curricular activities such as karate.

A number of studies that have evaluated CBT have shown consistent improvement in symptoms in depressed children and adolescents. One large study compared CBT interventions with nondirective supportive therapy and behavior therapy. About 70% of the adolescents in each condition improved, but the CBT intervention had the most rapid effect. Some studies have found CBT to be as effective as medication in alleviating symptoms of depression, and many professionals recommend starting with CBT (as opposed to medication) in children and adolescents with mild to moderate depression.

COGNITIVE BEHAVIOR THERAPY FOR ATTENTION-DEFICIT/ HYPERACTIVITY DISORDER

Betty was a 10-year-old girl who, according to her mom, had been "hyper since she was born!" Betty was diagnosed with attention-deficit/hyperactivity disorder at age 5 years, and although medication had improved her symptoms somewhat, she still experienced discipline problems at home and at school, struggled to complete her schoolwork, and had difficulty maintaining and making friends. Her symptoms were classic in that she had difficulty concentrating, had difficulty completing long or complex tasks, could not easily move from one task to another, had trouble following through on directions, and was always the "slowest one done" when asked to complete assigned work. As an adjunct to medication, Betty completed a course of CBT. Her therapy included the following:

- learning skills and steps that could guide her when completing a task or when in the midst of a complex social situation (e.g., Betty was taught to "take a breath" or "step back" before reacting and to consider alternative reactions to situations—rather than getting angry when she was frustrated because she could not complete tasks, Betty learned how to "use words" to convey her frustration which made her less likely to act in inappropriate, aggressive ways);
- learning calming techniques that helped her reduce her anger and frustration (e.g., one of these techniques included taking a break in the corner of the classroom and another allowed her to ask permission to take a walk to the front office so that she could "cool off" when she felt her behavior escalating);
- helping her parents and teachers learn ways of giving her feedback that rewarded her positive behaviors and corrected inappropriate behaviors; and
- applying study skills training and organizational help, such as learning how to take better notes and keep a calendar.

Betty's behavior improved considerably, but when she started high school, she came back to therapy. At this time, the therapist became less of a "teacher" and more of a "collaborator," emphasizing mutual problem-solving skills. Betty also learned how best to advocate for herself with her teachers and learned additional organizational strategies that helped her better manage the multiple tasks required of a high school student.

COGNITIVE BEHAVIOR THERAPY FOR OPPOSITIONAL DEFIANT DISORDER AND CONDUCT DISORDER

Benny was an 8-year-old boy who was described by his parents as constantly disobedient. He was easily annoyed and frequently aggravating to others. He frequently lost his temper, often over minor incidents such as not having the "right" cereal for his breakfast. He rarely finished his homework and never completed the chores that his parents asked him to do. With the exception of not completing his homework, he had few problems at school. In fact, when asked why he behaved this way at home, he replied, "Because my parents are always on my back."

Benny was diagnosed with oppositional defiant disorder. His behaviors are typical of children with this disorder in that he had patterns of negative attitudes, hostile behaviors, and disobedience. In contrast, children with conduct disorder engage in more severe acts of aggression that can cause physical harm to themselves and others. Benny's parents were worried he was heading in this direction because he had recently become more deceitful and had stolen money from a classmate's backpack. Benny's parents sought treatment with a psychologist who used a CBT approach that included teaching the parents how to alter their behavior to discourage Benny's oppositional behavior while simultaneously encouraging Benny's appropriate behaviors. Benny's therapist used a combination of meetings with the entire family, the parents with Benny, and Benny by himself. During the meetings with Benny, the therapist would have Benny practice more adaptive strategies that helped him develop a sense of mastery and success in situations he might encounter with family or friends. Within the safety of the therapeutic environment, Benny discovered he was capable of less aggressive behaviors. His therapist also understood that Benny's self-esteem needed to improve before he could make positive changes, and therefore increasing self-esteem was one of their goals. In terms of the parent–child relationship, Benny's therapist knew that patterns of harsh physical and verbal punishment can actually cause more aggressive and deviant behaviors, and he was afraid that Benny's parents' style of parenting was making matters worse. Thus, during his time with the parents, Benny's therapist helped them replace hard, punitive parenting techniques with gentler disciplining strategies.

Overall, CBT has been found to be quite effective in treating disruptive behavior disorders. Those that combine parent training and problem-solving-skills training in treating children are particularly effective. In fact, a combination of the two approaches has been shown to be more effective than either treatment alone, particularly for children 7 years of age and older. Common features of these programs include the following:

- a focus on the child's thought processes in his or her interpersonal relationships (e.g., during therapy the child is taught to solve interpersonal problems using a step-by-step process);
- an emphasis on improving prosocial behaviors through modeling or reinforcement;
- use of games, stories, and activities that teach better cognitive problem-solving skills and, as therapy progresses, increasing application of these skills to real-life situations at school and at home; and
- an active therapeutic approach in which the therapist models appropriate behaviors, teaches adaptive skills, and gives feedback for positive and negative behaviors.

COGNITIVE BEHAVIOR THERAPY FOR PHOBIAS

Nine-year-old Steve was overwhelmingly afraid of spiders. Until about a year ago, this did not present much of a problem. However, Steve really wanted to attend a summer sleep-away camp but was too afraid to go because he was afraid of seeing spiders in the woods and—even worse—in his tent. Steve's parents sought the expertise of a CBT therapist. Luckily, there is considerable support for the efficacy of using CBT approaches to treat phobias. During the early part of treatment, the therapist used a variety of techniques, all of which are well-established treatments. These included the following:

- *Graduated exposure* involved a process in which Steve faced the feared stimuli (the spider) for a sufficient period of time for him to become *habituated to* (i.e., used to) the feared object. The therapist started by teaching relaxation techniques and developing a *fear hierarchy* in which Steve had to list his fears about spiders from least scary (seeing a picture of a spider) to most scary (having a spider crawl on him). Once Steve was able to put himself in a relaxed state, the therapist presented items from the fear hierarchy (starting with the least feared items). She started by presenting these situations through imagery and then progressed to live situations that included seeing the spider and eventually having the spider crawl on him.
- *Modeling* appropriate behaviors involved the therapist modeling appropriate responses to the spider during the process of exposure therapy. These responses even included having Steve watch the spider crawl on her!
- *Reinforced practice* involved Steve practicing becoming comfortable with situations on the hierarchy and being reinforced for his behaviors. In addition, he was not forced to move up the hierarchy unless he was quite comfortable doing so.

Steve's spider phobia responded quite well to CBT. Within 16 weeks, he had gone from being enormously phobic of spiders, to having a spider crawl on his arm. While he did not enjoy the experience, he did tolerate it, and found himself capable of going to the summer camp he was so eager to attend.

COGNITIVE BEHAVIOR THERAPY
FOR OBSESSIVE–COMPULSIVE DISORDER

CBT is one of the more effective treatments for obsessive–compulsive disorder. It consists of educating the child about obsessive–compulsive disorder, teaching the child how to modify his thoughts to resist acting on obsessions and compulsions, and reinforcing the child for positive behaviors. One other approach, called *response prevention,* exposes the child to the situation that causes him anxiety while the compulsive ritual is prevented by helping the child resist the urge to perform it during the stressful condition. Another common technique, *imaginal exposure,* has the child imagine an anxiety-provoking condition for several minutes to the point of creating anxiety. At the same time, the child is not allowed to engage in thoughts or behaviors that would help her avoid the anxiety. Real-life exposure may also be used.

COGNITIVE BEHAVIOR THERAPY
FOR POSTTRAUMATIC STRESS DISORDER

CBT for posttraumatic stress disorder (PTSD) in adults has been rigorously studied and found to be effective in reducing PTSD symptoms. Although there are fewer studies using CBT to treat children with PTSD, a growing body of evidence supports its use in traumatized children. Some of the more rigorous studies have been completed in children who have been sexually abused, and CBT has been found to be as effective or more effective than any other approach.

CBT that involved both the parent and child was most effective, particularly with regard to improving aggressive and depressive symptoms. Therapy generally has a number of goals.

- The child's traumatic memories are discussed in detail so that they can be integrated into their autobiographical story. When this is done, the child is less likely to reexperience the symptoms.
- The child's misinterpretation of the event (e.g., thinking it was under his control) is explored and analyzed so that he does not feel responsible for the event and so that his sense of future threat is reduced.
- Poor coping strategies that exacerbate symptoms are eliminated.
- Misinterpretations of the event by the parents are identified and modified.
- Parents are used as collaborators in their child's treatments.

At the beginning of the therapeutic process, the focus is on engaging the child and parents in therapy and on normalizing the trauma. The therapist also helps the child and family gain a sense of normality by helping them see the need for scheduling positive activities and reassessing their faulty beliefs (e.g., "Our lives will never be the same." "I will never let my child out of my sight." "I can't ever trust anyone again."). Special interventions might be used, which can include the following:

- The therapist teaches the child (and sometimes the parents) relaxation techniques and good sleep habits.
- The therapist initiates *imaginal exposure* in which the child "relives" the trauma while feeling comfortable and relaxed. During this technique, the child is asked to talk about the trauma from the beginning until the point at which the child begins to feel anxious. During this procedure, the therapist

is helping the child realize he can tolerate the memories without necessarily feeling the anxiety.

- The therapist introduces *in vivo exposure* in which the child goes to the site of the trauma. For example, Connie was a 15-year-old who was involved in a car accident that left her mother in a coma for 2 weeks. Part of her therapy included going to the scene of the accident. Of note, this was done after Connie was feeling very comfortable with the therapist and after her mother had had a complete recovery.
- The therapist uses *cognitive restructuring,* which helps the child restructure any faulty beliefs about the trauma. For example, Connie felt that if she had not been playing with the radio controls in the car, her mother would not have been distracted, and the accident would not have happened. She also was afraid of driving in a car, thinking that she would be in another crash. As she reached driving age, she was fearful of getting her license because she thought she might cause another accident. Her therapist helped her appraise whether these beliefs were accurate and helped her correct her thinking about these issues.

Overall, CBT for PTSD is very effective. One of the most important components of treatment is a therapist who can apply these techniques in a flexible way. While treatment might be stressful at times, the stress should not be overwhelming, and you should notice at least gradual improvement with each week or month of treatment.

COGNITIVE BEHAVIOR THERAPY FOR ASPERGER'S SYNDROME, HIGH-FUNCTIONING AUTISM, AND PERVASIVE DEVELOPMENTAL DISORDER

Because CBT helps children focus on why they behave in certain ways, and the consequences of that behavior, CBT can be very useful for children and adolescents who have difficulty reading and interpreting social cues. CBT can be effective for children with Asperger's syndrome and pervasive developmental disorder who are treated in either group or individual formats. This therapy particularly helps children link emotions, responses, and consequences—links that are very difficult for children on this spectrum to make. Because doing this is difficult, this type of therapy is most useful in children who can cognitively make these links; therefore, it's most effective for adolescents and young adults who have mature abstract reasoning skills.

Judy, a 16-year-old with Asperger's syndrome, came to her therapy appointment confused because of the difficult week she had experienced. A few days before, she had written "Jenna sucks" and "Jenna should die" on the school's bathroom wall. Once it was discovered that she wrote this, she was suspended until she received a thorough psychological evaluation. The evaluation indicated that she was not dangerous but that she did not realize the implications of her actions. Judy was angry at Jenna (a friend) because Jenna had befriended a classmate, and Judy thought Jenna didn't like her anymore. Judy's therapist helped her to understand the links between her emotions, behavior, and consequences. Judy was able (with some effort) to articulate her anger at Jenna and also able to see how her anger may have been an overreaction to a situation that she had misinterpreted. Judy did not realize that writing aggressive statements on bathroom walls could get her into trouble. She also had limited awareness of other outcomes of her behaviors. For example, Judy did not realize that other kids might be less likely to associate with her because she had been suspended from school. Therapy also helped Judy learn better ways to manage these feelings in the future.

COGNITIVE BEHAVIOR THERAPY FOR EATING DISORDERS

The most effective treatment for bulimia is CBT, delivered either individually, in family therapy, or in combination. Although anorexia is a more difficult disorder to treat, CBT forms the basis for much of the treatment for anorexia. CBT therapists change eating behaviors by rewarding and modeling appropriate eating habits while helping patients change their distorted or rigid thinking patterns. Many patients hold themselves to perfectionist standards, which, because these standards cannot be met, cause the patient to be self-critical (e.g., "I'm so fat that anyone would think I am disgusting." "Everyone is looking at me because I look like a pig"). Treatment includes the following:

- establishing an appropriate eating plan that includes three meals a day plus snacks;
- keeping a diary of what the patient is eating, including the frequency, amount, thoughts and emotions connected with eating (and purging if that is an issue);
- using *response delays* such as waiting for a certain amount of time before engaging in purging or binging and, while waiting, engaging in an alternative activity such as calling a friend, reading a book, or listening to music;
- cognitively monitoring thoughts such as "my stomach is so fat" and, once the adolescent is aware of these thoughts and their frequency, working to evaluate and change these thoughts in therapy;
- using relaxation training and positive body imagery (i.e., imagining the positive aspects of a healthy body); and
- training the patient in problem-solving skills such as assertiveness and communication skills.

COGNITIVE BEHAVIOR THERAPY FOR BED-WETTING

Before starting any treatment for bed-wetting, the child should have a thorough evaluation to rule out medical issues. Once this has been done, behavioral treatments can be helpful. The most commonly used system is the *urine alarm system*. The device includes an absorbent sheet between two foil pads. When urine is absorbed in the sheet, the moisture activates an alarm that sounds until it is manually turned off. When the alarm sounds, the parents are taught to wake the child, at which point the child is taught to turn off the alarm and go to the bathroom to finish voiding. The seemingly simple system has been shown to be quite effective. In fact, treatment can change the patterns within a week, especially when the urine alarm system is combined with a technique called *dry bed training*. During this training, the therapist teaches the parents how to implement the following techniques at home:

- inhibiting urination,
- using positive reinforcement for correct urination (on the toilet),
- monitoring fluid intake,
- taking responsibility for accidents, and
- training in rapid awakening at home.

CONCLUDING THOUGHTS

As should be evident, CBT can be used to treat many disorders, ranging from mild problems to developmental difficulties to even more significant problems. It is a widely studied treatment and one that has been found to be quite effective. It can be used either alone or with other therapies and/or medication as part of a larger treatment plan. In addition to relieving current problems, there is research indicating that CBT also reduces the likelihood that a child or adolescent who is currently struggling with psychological problems will engage in additional problematic behaviors later in life. Overall, CBT is a well-validated therapy; however, as indicated in Chapter 2, the therapist's qualities and qualifications are also critical. Make sure you choose a therapist with whom you and your child feel comfortable. The best techniques are only as good as the therapist administering them.

CHAPTER 13

FAMILY THERAPY

Family therapy emphasizes the idea that a child lives and grows in relationship to others, particularly in relationship to members of his or her own family. There are many different family therapy approaches too numerous to list here. However, nearly all of the approaches assume that the child's "problem" (whatever it might be) does not just reside with the child but is at least in part determined by variables in the larger family system. Unlike most of the other therapies discussed in this book, which focus on what is happening to the child as an individual, family therapists work with the entire family system to heal problematic relationships and to mobilize family resources to help the child with the presenting problem and the family. One of the aims of this therapy is to help family members discover the role they play within the family's social structure. Another goal is to help family members communicate better with one another and to learn new ways of preventing or resolving conflicts. This not only helps the child who is symptomatic but also benefits the rest of the family.

In family therapy, a child's personality—how he thinks, feels, and acts—is seen as a result of the complicated interactions and relationships that occur in the family. Within the family system, there are *subsystems,* such as the *marital subsystem* (the mom and dad) and the *sibling subsystem* (the children). How these subsystems interact can result in a family being balanced or not, but many events and situations can cause even the best families to become imbalanced. For example, when Luke was in third grade, his dad lost his job. Luke's parents started fighting about money all of the time—to the point that Luke was too anxious to sleep at night. Within a few months, Luke started performing poorly at school and started getting into fights on the school bus. Although the initial referral was for Luke to get therapy to help him with his aggressive behaviors, the therapist soon realized that Luke's behavior was just a symptom of the stress within the family. Even after his father started working again, the family system failed to regain its stability. Poor communication strategies had developed; resentments had built up; and Luke's behavior was disturbing to both his parents and his 12-year-old sister, who had recently started becoming truant from school. Family therapy was a place in which all of these problems could be addressed at the same time. Although a therapist might be tempted to focus just on Luke's aggressive behavior and recent school failure, using this therapeutic process to address problems with communication between the parents, help the parents learn better parenting skills to address their child's recent misbehaviors, and strengthen the family bond was a much more powerful way to help every member of the family.

Many different mental health professionals can provide family therapy, but it is usually provided by therapists who have expertise in this area. They are often referred to as *marriage and family therapists.* Many psychologists, psychiatrists, social workers, and other mental health experts have training in this area. Before engaging in treatment with a professional, it is important to ask him or her about qualifications. Questions can include: Do you have additional training in family therapy? How many families have you treated? What types of problems have you successfully treated? It is important to find a licensed mental health professional. Many marriage and family therapists are credentialed by the American Association for Marriage and Family Therapy, which sets specific criteria for eligibility. However, there are many qualified licensed professionals who are not members of the American Association of Marriage and Family Therapy, so it is not crucial that you find a professional with this qualification.

It is not uncommon for a family to participate in family therapy along with other types of mental health treatment. For example, Luke's father realized that he had been depressed since he lost his job, and even though life was looking better, he didn't feel like himself. He started attending individual therapy along with family therapy. In addition, Luke started talking to the guidance counselor at school about his aggressive behavior. These additional therapies were actually quite helpful adjuncts to the family therapy process.

During the process of family therapy, the therapist often focuses on one or more of the following areas:

- providing family members with information about how families generally function and particularly how their own family functions,
- looking at the problem not as an individual problem but as one that focuses on the family as a whole,
- teaching better communication skills,
- helping the family identify areas of conflicts and situations that may make certain family members anxious or angry,
- helping all family members to feel better about themselves and realize they are not alone, and
- using the strengths within the family to help all family members handle their problems.

Family therapy is often a short-term treatment, but the number of sessions varies depending on how severe the problems are and how willing the family members are to engage in treatment. Not all family members will attend each session. At the beginning of treatment, the family and therapist set goals, and the therapist determines who needs to attend particular sessions. For example, if the problem is due to a lack of communication between the parents, the therapist might have the parents come in for sessions twice a month. The children may come alone one other time during the month, and the entire family will convene once during the month. There are no hard-and-fast rules for scheduling family therapy appointments, so it is most important to work with a qualified therapist you trust.

WHO CAN BENEFIT FROM FAMILY THERAPY?

Family therapy can be used to treat a wide range of issues, and there are a number of studies showing its effectiveness in treating children with oppositional behaviors, adolescent acting out, anxiety, substance use, eating disorders, and school problems. Most referrals for family therapy fall into one of the following categories:

- children who are having problems in school because of learning, emotional, or behavioral problems;
- adolescent conflicts with parents;
- conflicts within the parent's relationship;
- conflicts within the sibling relationships;
- grief, loss, and trauma;
- chronic mental health or physical health problems that have not been responsive to other forms of treatment; and
- one family member's chronic illness, such as alcoholism, severe depression, or schizophrenia.

Just because your particular problem doesn't fall into one of the listed categories doesn't mean your family cannot benefit from family therapy. In fact, family therapy can also be useful before problems begin. For example, a man and woman with children from previous marriages may go into family therapy before they get married so that the children and parents can learn to live with one another in the best way possible.

WHAT IS THE TYPICAL COURSE OF TREATMENT IN FAMILY THERAPY?

Family therapists have different ways of approaching the family system, and there are many valid ways of doing this. Some therapists prefer to meet first with the parents, whereas others want to meet initially with the entire family. During the initial sessions, the therapist focuses on how family members interact with one another: What kinds of information do family members share? Who does most of the talking? How do family members talk to one another? Are certain family members allied with one another in a way that excludes other family members? After the therapist has a better understanding of the situation, she may make start to make interventions to change the way family members interact. The therapist may have family members reenact different scenarios using more appropriate communication techniques. She may have family members complete different homework assignments that could include having family members spend time with one another. For example, if an adolescent son and his father have had difficulty communicating, the therapist may tell them to do something together that they both enjoy, such as fishing, and then report back what the experience was like. The therapist may have family members role-play other family members. For example, the adolescent son might be asked to play the role of dad during a fight while the father is asked to play the role of his adolescent son. In this instance, actually having to be in the other person's shoes can help family members gain empathy and perspective.

WHAT TYPES OF CHILDHOOD DISORDERS HAVE BEEN SHOWN TO BE TREATED EFFECTIVELY BY FAMILY THERAPY?

Children with a wide variety of disorders can be helped by family therapy, although the type of therapeutic approach, the frequency of sessions, and the configuration of treatment (i.e., whether the parents sometimes attend without the children) vary according to the needs of the family and the therapist's approach. Family treatment has been well researched in a number of specific disorders, and what follows are highlights of the disorders that have been most effectively treated with family therapy techniques.

Attention-Deficit/Hyperactivity Disorder

When a child struggles with attention-deficit/hyperactivity disorder (ADHD), it is not uncommon for the entire family to struggle as well. Children with ADHD have problems inhibiting their impulses, cannot stop what they are doing when it is time to stop, and do not pay attention when it is time to focus. These types of behaviors occur many times on a daily basis within the family system. For example, Carl was a 7-year-old boy who never sat at the table for dinner because he couldn't sit still. He could not complete his homework unless his parents yelled at him the entire time. His older sister was starting to develop symptoms of anxiety because, as she said, "The family is arguing about things all the time!" Family therapy helped Carl's parents learn better strategies for managing his behavior. Through the course of therapy, Carl learned he was not "bad" but that he learned and behaved differently from his sister. His sister learned how to better communicate her feelings with the rest of the family.

Within the context of family therapy, role playing was used to let family members show each other how they each see the other members. Since people with ADHD are poor at realizing the effect their behavior has on others, watching others play them can help them truly see the types of behaviors that are causing other family members to be distressed. Sometimes it is not that the child with ADHD is unwilling to change but that the child is not even aware of what he needs to change. These types of interventions can be quite helpful in this regard. Although it is difficult to predict what strategies will work best with what particular families, the most effective techniques include the following:

- teaching the parents better ways to manage their child's behavior using behavior management techniques,
- helping parents structure and organize the child's environment in a way that will help him focus better and decrease problem behaviors, and
- helping the child see the effect of his own behavior on other family members.

Disruptive Behavior Disorders

Oppositional defiant disorder and conduct disorder are disorders in which the child consistently defies authority, possesses a strong need for control, and displays a pattern of negativistic behavior. Research has shown that oppositional behaviors are more prevalent when there are problems in the home, most particularly when there is too much or too little structure in the home. When the environment is too structured, the parenting style is generally rigid and inflexible, and the child is often micromanaged. Children and adolescents react to this by becoming oppositional and defiant. In contrast, a home life that lacks structure can also create oppositional behaviors because this type of parenting style tends to be one in which the parents give in to the child's demands while providing few consequences for misbehaviors. In addition, oppositional behaviors and conduct problems can be a reaction to stress within the marital relationship.

207

For example, when parents are having difficulty getting along, they disagree on parenting style, which makes it hard for them to be successful in changing their child's behavior.

Because of these reasons, family therapy is one of the most successful ways of treating disruptive behaviors. Therapy can be helpful in many ways, including the following:

- helping the family resolve family difficulties;
- providing parents with techniques for avoiding conflict, such as walking away from a fight, acting rationally when the child seems desperate for a fight, and staying calm and unemotional in emotionally laden situations; and
- learning to use effective consequences, including developing and setting clear rules and consequences and removing reinforcers (unless they are earned).

A few specialized treatments found to be effective in treating children with conduct disorders also have a family therapy component. Two of the most effective treatments are (a) *parent management training*, a program that teaches parents to change their child's behavior by improving parent–child interactions and communication and enhancing parenting skills such as monitoring and supervising their child's behavior; and (b) *multisystemic therapy*, a very intensive family and community-based approach in which treatment is carried out with the child's family, school personnel, peers, and even the juvenile justice system if necessary. This therapy draws from many different approaches, including marital therapy, substance abuse treatment, and special education services, as needed.

Overall, there have been many advances in treating oppositional defiant disorder and conduct disorder, although much work remains to be done. In terms of outcome, the degree of success or failure depends in a large part on the severity of the child's problems.

Children who have mild to moderate problems from middle-class homes have the best rates of successful treatment, whereas children from highly chaotic homes who are also from poor neighborhoods have the poorest rates of success.

Alcohol and Drug Abuse

Adolescent drug and alcohol use is a complicated problem, and treatments to address it are typically multifaceted. In seeking treatment for an adolescent's substance abuse, it is very important to find clinicians who have experience in this area because this is a specific population that needs specialized treatment. Most treatment programs incorporate some type of family therapy into substance abuse treatment. Family therapy can be helpful in using the family's strengths and resources to help the abuser. It can also help families become aware of their own needs; siblings in the family may find their needs ignored when their brother or sister moves from one crisis to another, and parents may find themselves constantly arguing over the stress that has been created in the family.

Unfortunately, treatment for substance use disorders can be somewhat disappointing because about half of adolescents receiving treatment for substance use disorders will relapse within the first 3 months following treatment. However, the more promising treatments involve the systems that affect the adolescent—particularly the family system. Similar to the types of strategies mentioned previously in oppositional defiant disorder and conduct disorder, family-based approaches for substance use disorder attempt to do the following:

- decrease negative interactions between family members,
- improve communication between family members, and
- develop better problem-solving skills that address areas of conflict.

Multisystemic therapy (mentioned previously) is especially effective because it involves the family, peer relationships, school, and community. In general, the intensity of treatment will depend on the level of use and the adolescent's home environment. Adolescents who have stable home environments with low to moderate levels of use can be treated well with outpatient therapy, whereas adolescents with more severe abuse (and with comorbid psychological issues such as bipolar disorder or depression) may need an inpatient or residential setting.

Eating Disorders

It is not surprising that family therapy is used as a technique for treating eating disorders such as anorexia and bulimia because families are often intimately involved in the development of eating disorders. Research has also shown that families are quite involved in maintaining the behaviors associated with these disorders. Because these disorders can be difficult to treat, often a multidimensional approach is used that incorporates individual therapy, behavioral management techniques, family therapy, and medical treatment. Aspects of the family therapy component include the following:

- educating the family members on the disorder,
- helping family members see their role in the maintenance of the behaviors,
- providing insight to the family members with regard to dysfunctional family patterns,
- helping adolescents find ways to achieve age-appropriate separation because many adolescents with eating disorders have trouble making the transition to young adulthood,
- enhancing communication between family members,

- helping family members better express their personal needs and feelings more clearly, and
- helping family members understand their "relationship" with food.

Overall, family involvement is usually a key component of the treatment package for eating disorders. This is especially true if the adolescent is still a minor and if she still resides with her family of origin.

Anxiety

As indicated in Chapter 13, a number of cognitive behavior treatments are effective for treating anxiety disorders. However, anxiety often occurs in families in which multiple family members are anxious or in the context of high-conflict family relationships that increase anxious symptoms. When a child becomes anxious, it can change the parent's perception of what the child is capable of doing.

For example, Kenny was a 7-year-old who developed an anxiety disorder. The more anxious he seemed, the more his parents "jumped through hoops" to keep him calm. This meant keeping him home from school if he was having a bad day or serving him dinner in bed if he was too nervous to leave his room. Addressing his symptoms in the context of the family relationship resulted in lasting changes for him and for the family. During the therapy, the therapist worked on the following areas, which are areas typically covered when treating anxiety in family therapy:

- managing emotions (both Kenny's and his parents'),
- exploring interactions within the family system,
- increasing communication skills, and
- helping his parents develop better problem-solving skills in managing Kenny's behavior.

Given the important role of the family in anxiety and obsessive–compulsive disorder, treatments for anxiety and obsessive–compulsive disorder have increasingly emphasized family therapy components. Recent research has shown this to be quite effective in treating children with these difficulties.

Phobias

Phobias can be effectively treated with various cognitive behavior approaches, such as exposure therapy, but phobias can cause major problems within the family system in that they can limit the activities a family can do together. Parents describe living with a child with a phobia as "walking on eggshells" to avoid a scene that can be caused by the phobia. Because of this, family therapy can help family members develop better ways of coping with the phobic behaviors. In addition, family members often attend therapy sessions so that they can serve as a coach when the child practices exposure therapy (being exposed ever so slowly to the feared object).

CONCLUDING THOUGHTS

Although this chapter provides only a brief synopsis of family therapy, I hope it has given you a taste for how it can be applied to a variety of childhood disorders. Family therapy is frequently used in conjunction with other therapeutic approaches. For example, psychodynamic therapists may use family therapy techniques with some of their cases as deemed necessary. Although most child psychologists have had some form of training in family therapy, only some actually specialize in this approach. When a qualified professional provides family therapy, it can have very positive results, either as the sole treatment or as an adjunct to other forms of treatment.

CHAPTER 14

SCHOOL-BASED SERVICES

When children are struggling with psychological or learning issues, services provided at their school may be a key ingredient in treatment. For example, Juan was a hyperactive third grader who was recently diagnosed with attention-deficit/hyperactivity disorder. His doctor prescribed medication, which seemed to be working well, and Juan and his parents attended weekly family therapy sessions to learn ways of managing his behavior at home. Even though the family had made progress in the home environment, Juan was still struggling at school. The medication caused him to be less hyperactive, but he still could not complete his written work. He was disorganized, had difficulty getting started on tasks, and didn't know how to study for tests. In addition to the treatments provided outside of school, it was recommended that Juan get in-school services. In his case, he received resource-room support for help with organization and study skills and accommodations, such as having tasks broken down into smaller components. In addition, he was seated at the front of the class near the teacher, given frequent breaks, and given frequent feedback from his teacher. He also received occupational therapy to remediate his problems with handwriting. These school services improved Juan's skills considerably at school; this led him to feeling better about himself in general, which resulted in positive behaviors outside of the school environment.

Juan received services under an individual educational plan (IEP). An IEP is developed when a child is found to be eligible for special education services. It provides services and accommodations that will help your child participate in the general curriculum. In Juan's case, it was determined that without accommodations such as those listed in the preceding paragraph and without special services in handwriting and study skills, he would not be able to access the curriculum that other students his age without disabilities were learning. The IEP addresses problems in academics but also other concerns. The Individuals With Disabilities Education Act (IDEA) is the federal law that defines a child's right to special services. To be eligible for special education services, a child must have a disability recognized by IDEA and because of the disability require specially designed instruction of specialized services. The disability categories specified in IDEA include

- a specific learning disability in a subject such as reading, math, or written expression;
- autism or pervasive developmental disorder;
- mental retardation;
- emotional disturbances, such as depression or anxiety;
- speech and language disorders;
- traumatic brain injury;
- severe orthopedic impairment, such as cerebral palsy or amputation;
- "other health impairment," which can include medical disabilities (multiple sclerosis, diabetes, eating disorders) and attention-deficit/hyperactivity disorder; and
- hearing or vision impairment.

These are the federal guidelines, but be sure to check with your state guidelines because they may vary. State laws can provide additional rights to children, but they cannot go below the level of protection set forth in IDEA. For example, in many states, developmental delays for children ages 3 to 9 years are considered disabilities even though the child does not meet a disability in any of the other previously mentioned areas.

If you think your child needs services at school, it is important to have a thorough evaluation completed either through the school district or through a private evaluator. There are advantages and disadvantages to pursuing either one, and many parents decide to do a combination of the two. In other words, they may ask the school to evaluate some aspects of their child's functioning and a private evaluator to look at other aspects of functioning. Once an evaluation has been completed, the school will call a meeting to discuss the results and recommendations. The meeting must include the parents, a regular education teacher, a special education teacher (if your child is already getting services), a staff person from the school district who is familiar with the resources in the system, and a school staff person who can interpret the results of the evaluation. Very often this staff person is the school psychologist. Once a child turns 14 years of age, the child must be invited to attend the meeting (although the child does not always come). You can bring other people to the meeting as well. For example, if your child has been depressed and has been working with a psychologist, you may want to invite the psychologist to the meeting. During this meeting, the team will determine whether your child meets criteria for an IEP. You, as the parent or guardian, may reject or accept the findings of the meeting. You can reject the findings whether they qualify or do not qualify for services. If you reject the findings of the IEP, you should state your concerns in writing and send them to your child's school district. Your state's law may specify the amount of time you have to respond

What Is a Section 504 Plan?

A *Section 504 plan* applies to children who have learning, emotional, or performance weaknesses that do not meet the criteria for an IEP. A 504 plan is not considered special education but is an accommodation plan that states the child may need modifications to the curriculum to meet his or her needs. Accommodations can include extra time on tests, preferential seating, or breaking up tasks into smaller components. Even slight modifications such as sitting in the front of the room can have a significant effect on a child's learning. For some children, a 504 plan is enough to support their learning and emotional needs. Requirements for 504 plans vary by state, so it's important to check your state's guidelines before determining whether an IEP or 504 plan is right for your child.

What Is Early Intervention?

Early intervention is a comprehensive, multidisciplinary system of care that provides services for infants and toddlers with disabilities. Children younger than 3 years of age who have developmental delays or a diagnosable disorder may be eligible for early intervention services. These free services provide intensive support in any area of need, including physical development, speech therapy, occupational therapy, psychological services, audiological services, social work, counseling, family training, and home visits. Each state is provided grants from the federal government to provide services to infants and toddlers with disabilities. The state establishes criteria for eligibility within the parameters set by the federal government, so it is important to check with your local school system to see who can help you determine whether your child is eligible for services.

to the school in writing, and it is a good idea to check on this soon after the meeting.

WHAT TYPES OF PROBLEMS CAN BE EFFECTIVELY TREATED IN THE SCHOOL SETTING?

Many if not most psychological and learning issues can, at least in part, be addressed within the school environment. After all, school is the place where children spend most of their waking hours. What follows are highlights of the disorders that are more commonly and successfully treated with school interventions. Keep in mind this is not meant to be an exhaustive list. If you think your child is in need of services, don't be afraid to talk with your child's principal, guidance counselor, or school psychologist. They can help you to determine whether your child might need further evaluation or some type of intervention. However, you should remember that if their assessment of the problem doesn't feel right to you, you should trust your judgment and seek a second opinion from a private professional. Similarly, if you have first consulted with a private professional who stated that your child should be "completely fine" at school but you think otherwise, seek a second opinion from the school psychologist. No professional is perfect, and when in doubt, seek a second opinion.

Attention-Deficit/Hyperactivity Disorder

There is a wealth of research data showing that the use of behavioral techniques in the classroom can help treat academic performance problems in children with attention-deficit/hyperactivity disorder. Interventions such as manipulating the curriculum, changing the environment, and peer tutoring have all been found to be effective. Other interventions such as reducing task length, "chunking" tasks into smaller units, and setting specific and reasonable goals are also helpful. Teaching

217

styles play a role; vibrant, enthusiastic teachers who work hard to engage children and allow children to participate in teaching increase the child's attention. The use of written, displayed schedules and setting timers for task limits may further benefit these children.

Conduct Problems

There are a number of effective approaches that are used within the classroom for children with conduct problems such as oppositional defiant disorder and conduct disorder. Many of these approaches include some sort of behavioral token system in which the child earns points or tokens for good behavior. In addition to token rewards, other elements of successful classroom management of conduct problems include

- establishment of clear rules and directions;
- use of instructional materials that pace the student's academic progress at his or her own rate;
- providing positive and corrective feedback; and
- use of punishment techniques, such as time outs, reprimands, and loss of privileges for disruptive behaviors that cannot be ignored.

Learning Disabilities

Learning disabilities such as dyslexia, math disorder, and disorder of written expression are best treated within the school setting. Although psychologists in private practice (and school psychologists as well) can be very helpful in treating the associated symptoms of learning disabilities such as depression, anxiety, and poor self-esteem, the treatment really needs to include specific remediation in areas of academic functioning within the school environment.

For example, if your child has a reading disability or dyslexia, the optimal teaching approach is the use of a multisensory, sequential, phonics-based approach to teaching reading. The three most commonly used (and most widely researched) approaches are the Orton Gillingham, the Lindamood Bell, and the Wilson methods. These approaches are similar to each other, and most children with reading difficulties will respond to any one of them. If it is determined that your child has a reading disability, you should request special education services for reading. Your school may not have a certified specialist in one of the previously mentioned approaches, and if the school doesn't, you may need to advocate for these services. This may require the school to find someone who works outside of the school district. The intensity of the intervention is important, and most children require at least two to three sessions per week (for 45 minutes each). Sometimes the intensity of the services is not adequate at school, and parents opt to supplement the school services with private tutoring. Other types of accommodations that are frequently needed in children with dyslexia include

- extra time on tests,
- advance notice of large reading assignments,
- books on tape,
- use of spell-checking devices,
- writing tutoring because many students with dyslexia have trouble with written expression,
- tutoring in organizational and executive function skills because many children with learning disabilities struggle in this area, and
- tutoring in reading comprehension strategies.

If your child has a math disorder, the standard treatment is tutoring in mathematics. There are no standard treatments for math problems as there are for reading disabilities mainly because problems in math can be due to a number of issues. For example, some children have problems with math because they have problems with visual–spatial confusion, whereas other children have trouble because they do not understand the underlying concepts, and still others have difficulty because they have trouble remembering basic math facts and procedures. Some children have problems in multiple areas. Thus, the tutoring needs to focus on the particular area(s) of difficulty. To determine this, a comprehensive battery of tests is required so that the tutoring approach can be individually tailored to the child's needs. Other approaches that are helpful include

- use of a calculator (for older students) to help the child focus on the conceptual task at hand rather than the computational underpinnings;
- use of concrete materials to teach math concepts;
- providing "written recipes" for complex tasks such as dividing fractions or algebraic equations;
- learning concepts such as evaluating what operation is required to complete the problem, evaluating essential and nonessential information (particularly in story problems), and estimating and checking answers;
- occupational therapy for students who have significant problems with visual–motor processing; and
- requesting special education services in math if your child has a documented learning disability in math.

If your child has been diagnosed with a disorder of written expression, the standard treatment is tutoring in writing skills. Similar to what was mentioned previously with regard to math, there is no one-size-fits-all approach to writing tutoring. Some children need help with the actual motor task of writing (and would be treated with occupational therapy), whereas other students have more difficulty organizing their thoughts or generating a written narrative. Some students have both, and it is important to get a thorough evaluation so you have a good idea of what kind of remediation will be most helpful. Writing tutoring can focus on things such as organizing ideas, grammar, correct spelling, learning how to use outlines, proofreading, and how to generate an interesting narrative. Other recommendations can include

- allowing the child to take oral exams when feasible;
- allowing the child to have additional time for tests;
- using the computer for writing tasks;
- obtaining notes from the teacher (so that the student does not have to concentrate on taking notes) or audiotaping classes;
- modification of written assignments as needed, such as shortening the length of the assignment; and
- special education services for writing.

Nonverbal Learning Disorder or Asperger's Syndrome

The deficits seen in children with nonverbal learning disorder or Asperger's syndrome generally fall into one of the following categories: problems processing nonverbal information, social skills deficits, and motor coordination problems. There is great variation in children with nonverbal learning disorders and Asperger's syndrome, and although some need no school support, others need a very specialized level of support. There are a number of great books and websites that cover this issue in detail (see the Additional Resources section in this book), but school-based treatment can include

- tutoring in specific areas of learning such as reading comprehension, writing, or math when needed;
- tutoring in executive function and organizational and study skills;

- tailoring the classroom environment, such as smaller class size or the availability of a classroom aide;
- speech and language therapy that address problems with the pragmatic (or social) aspects of language;
- participation in a social skills group where children learn ways to appropriately interact with their peers; and
- occupational therapy for difficulties with motor functioning.

Autism and Pervasive Development Disorder

Most children with autism and pervasive development disorder require some level of school support, and some may need considerable support, such as a specialized classroom setting. Usually the best approach

My Child Has Autism. Would He Be Better Off in a Specialized Classroom or in a Regular Classroom With Additional Support?

The answer to this question really depends on the individual child. Generally, if your child is performing at or near grade level and has few behavior problems (e.g., extreme hyperactivity or aggression), he could probably benefit from a regular classroom setting. Depending on the number of students in the class, you may want to request a classroom aide who can offer continuous support during the day. I generally recommend that parents directly observe the different classroom settings because I find that most parents know whether their child could cope in a particular classroom environment. It is fortunate that you don't have to make that decision on your own because you will have the support of school personnel. But you may know—once you take a look at the other children in the classroom—whether you can imagine your child being successful in that environment. Your feedback can be quite helpful in determining the best environment for your child. Consulting a private psychologist with a specialty in autism can also provide a helpful second opinion.

is a multifaceted one, and the public school system may be the place where the services are coordinated. One specialized approach for children with autism is applied behavior analysis. This is a type of treatment that is based on behavioral principles of psychology, such as reinforcing appropriate behaviors, ignoring inappropriate ones, and targeting specific behaviors. Applied behavior analysis generally focuses on increasing adaptive prosocial behaviors and reducing maladaptive behaviors. It can be used to teach new skills, to generalize behaviors to other settings, and to reduce inappropriate behaviors such as self-injurious behaviors. Another treatment approach that has been widely researched and found to be effective is the Treatment and Education of Autistic and Related Communication-Handicapped Children program (TEACH), which emphasizes visual structure and organization of the environment and learning materials. This program uses a child's visual, mechanical, and rote memory skills (which are often relative strengths for children with autism) to develop language, cognitive, and social skills. Other school-based services could include

- a structured classroom environment for children with pervasive development disorder and autism,
- allied support services such as occupational therapy or speech therapy,
- social skills training,
- a one-to-one aide oftentimes trained in applied behavior analysis, and
- after-school and/or home-based services that are paid for by the school district.

Depression, Anxiety, and Other Psychological Concerns

These types of issues are often treated outside of the school environment, but there are times that school services are useful. For example, Maria was a 16-year-old high school student who was diagnosed with

My Child Attends Private School and Was Just Diagnosed With a Reading Disability. Can I Expect the Private School to Provide Services for Her?

The answer to this question depends on the school, and your first stop should be to the child's advisor or guidance counselor. An increasing number of private schools offer specialized support in specific subjects such as reading, writing, and math. Your school may also offer support in study skills and may be happy to accommodate certain requests such as extra time on tests or preferential seating. Your child has presumably received a comprehensive evaluation (because she was diagnosed with a learning disability). I would recommend sharing the results of the evaluation with the school, which can then determine what types of services are available. If your school does not provide services, you can opt to have tutoring occur after school, and you should know that private schools are not required to address learning issues as public schools are.

The Neuropsychologist Who Diagnosed my Child With ADHD Recommended we Share the Complete Results With the School, but my Husband Wants to Only Share the Diagnosis and Recommendations. *What Should I do?*

I generally suggest sharing all the results with the school, whether the school is private or public. Parents are understandably nervous about this, but schools see dozens of these reports every year and know how to interpret these data. I find that sometimes schools are suspicious when they receive a one-page synopsis of the findings and often would not implement services without seeing the actual data. There are exceptions to this rule; if the evaluation seems to be invalid (in other words, if the evaluation doesn't fit with your experience of your child) or if there is personal family information that the school doesn't need to know, you are well within your bounds not to share the information or to ask for the personal information to be deleted from the version of the report that will be shared with the school.

depression. At first she was able to cope with her symptoms at school (although she frequently spent the rest of her time in bed), but when her depression worsened and started to interfere with her ability to perform in school, support services were put in place for her. These included giving her extensions on her homework, a reduced course load, and frequent check-ins with the school psychologist. These types of problems are generally not covered under an IEP because there typically is not a need to change the curriculum for children who are feeling depressed or anxious. However, services might be covered under a 504 plan. This was the case for Maria, whose 504 plan included the accommodations listed previously.

CONCLUDING THOUGHTS

Your local school system can provide a wealth of support for your child, but sometimes you may need to be the catalyst that makes the services "happen." You are your child's best advocate, and although most of the time schools will provide the appropriate services, this is not always the case. If you feel your child isn't getting what he or she needs at school, isn't making appropriate progress, or is coming home hating school, something is wrong, and you should ask for an evaluation or—if your child has been recently evaluated—find out if the services that are supposed to be in place are actually being implemented. If your school does not think an evaluation is necessary but you do, you should consider pursuing a private evaluation. The good news is that if services are deemed necessary, they are free and provided in the context of your child's school day. Furthermore, these services may be the key to putting your child on the road to success.

CHAPTER 15

OTHER TREATMENT OPTIONS

Thus far in this book, I have reviewed psychological treatments that are available to treat different types of problems, but those are not the only treatments available. Though many childhood psychological disorders respond to therapy alone, some children need additional services. The most common adjunct treatment is medication, but depending on your child's problem, other forms of therapy might be indicated. These can include *occupational therapy,* which treats fine and gross motor skills and general self-help skills; *physical therapy,* which is used to treat gross motor skills such as balance, coordination, and muscle strength; and *speech and language therapy,* which treats a child's ability to use language, understand language, and speak clearly. Depending on your child's particular issue, one or more of these treatments may be helpful, either with psychotherapy or in place of it.

MEDICATION

No treatment approach is quite as anxiety provoking as medication, even though it can be extremely helpful when appropriately prescribed. You may find yourself baffled by the range and possibilities of medications, and the answers to your questions are far beyond the scope of this book. Luckily, the resources in the appendix to this book that can provide you with more information. Deciding to use medication to address your child's problems is a big step, and it is normal to have many questions. I strongly advise that you insist on getting satisfactory answers from your child's prescribing physician. Generally, though, medications fall into specific categories, discussed next.

Medications Used to Treat Attention-Deficit/ Hyperactivity Disorder

As you may remember from Chapter 4, the best interventions for attention-deficit/hyperactivity disorder (ADHD) involve a combination of treatments, and this combination often includes medication. Using medication to treat ADHD has been the subject of debate for many years, but despite the controversy, medication is the most effective treatment for managing symptoms of ADHD. The most commonly prescribed medications are *stimulants,* drugs that stimulate the part of the brain that is understimulated in children with ADHD by affecting neurotransmitters (particularly dopamine). Neurotransmitters allow brain cells (or *neurons*) to communicate with one another, and these medications increase the communication signal between these cells. A doctor can choose from a number of stimulant medications, and each works a bit differently in the brain. Thus, you may find that one stimulant medication works quite well, whereas another one does not. The most commonly prescribed stimulant is methylphenidate, and the brand names include Ritalin, Concerta, Metadate, Daytrana, Adderall, Dexedrine, Focalin, and Methylin. Strattera was the first non-stimulant medication for ADHD, and it has been found to be effective for many children. Many studies have documented positive effects

> **What Are the Most Common Side Effects**
> **From Stimulant Medications?**
>
> The most common side effects are loss of appetite and difficulty sleeping, but other side effects can include dizziness, irritability, moodiness, and possible growth problems (i.e., slower growth rate).

of these medications on children's social interactions, cooperation, aggressive behaviors, academic productivity, and attention.

Medications Used to Treat Depression

As you might guess, the class of drugs known as *antidepressants* is used to treat depression in children, but some have also been found to help children and adolescents with ADHD, anxiety disorders, and bed-wetting. In other words, don't be surprised if your doctor prescribes an antidepressant even though your child is not depressed. The most commonly used antidepressants are the *selective serotonin reuptake inhibitors*. These are usually the first-line intervention for children with moderate to severe depression and are named for the effect the drugs have on serotonin, a brain chemical. This class of drugs includes Prozac, Paxil, Celexa, Zoloft, Lexapro, and Luvox. Another class of antidepressants is *tricyclics*. They get their name from the fact that the chemical structure of the drugs has three rings (i.e., tricycles). These drugs include Elavil, Tofranil, Norpramin, Pamelor, Anafranil and Vivactyl. A final class of antidepressants includes the *atypical antidepressants,* such as Wellbutrin, Effexor, Remeron, Cymbalta, and Trazodone. They are referred to as *atypical* because their chemical structures and effect on brain chemistry are different from the other drugs.

What Are the Most Common Side Effects From Antidepressants?

Sometimes children can become agitated, have stomach upset, headaches, changes in appetite, sleep problems, and irritability. Some children will have emotional and behavioral side effects, such as a worsening of depression or increased anxiety. It is very important to stay in close contact with your doctor and to report any possible side effects immediately.

Mood Stabilizing Medications

Mood stabilizing medications are used, unsurprisingly, to stabilize one's mood. For example, this class of drugs can help stabilize the rapidly changing mood swings and aggressiveness in a child with bipolar disorder. Unfortunately, with the use of these medications in children is very understudied. Many children with bipolar disorder are given multiple medications, but there is currently little data showing the effectiveness of mood stabilizers on children's unstable moods. Despite this, these medications are used to address manic symptoms and mood instability in children because adults with mood instability are helped by using these drugs. The most commonly used mood stabilizing medication is lithium but other drugs such as Tegretol, Trileptal, Depakote, Neurontin, Lamictal, and Topamax are also frequently prescribed. Some of these drugs were developed to treat other conditions. For example, Tegretol is actually an anticonvulsant drug used to treat epilepsy, but it can also work as a mood stabilizer because it reduces the firing of nerve impulses in the brain. Side effects of these medications can be significant and can include nausea, upset stomach, sleepiness, tremor, and weight gain. Long-term effects can include thyroid problems and kidney damage, so it is important for your child's health to be closely monitored while on these medications.

Medications Used to Treat Anxiety Disorders

These medications are referred to as *anxiolytics,* and they are used to treat symptoms of panic, anxiety, nervousness, and worry. Often antidepressants are first used to treat anxiety disorders, but some-times, particularly when the anxiety is severe, your doctor may pre-scribe a *benzodiazepine* (e.g., Valium, Klonopin, Xanax). These drugs typically have a sedating effect on the nervous system and can cause your child to be drowsy or sleepy. There are no serious side effects from this class of drugs (when used correctly), but children can build up a tolerance for the drugs, so more of a drug may be required to reduce the symptoms, and there is a small potential risk of dependency. Thus, your doctor will likely be quite cautious in prescribing these medications.

Medications Used to Treat Psychosis

This class of drugs, called *antipsychotics,* is used to treat psychotic symptoms in children, but it is also used to treat other disorders such as mood instability, agitation, and severe aggression. These drugs include Risperdal, Zyprexa, Seroquel, Abilify, and Geodone. These medications have significant side effects and are rarely the first choice of any medical doctor unless the symptoms are clearly due to bipolar disorder, schizophrenia, or other psychotic illness. The most common side effects are weight gain, sleepiness, and increased appetite, but more severe (and sometimes) lifelong side effects can occur, which can include repetitive movements such as lip smacking or grimacing.

The various medications that are used to treat psychological symptoms can dramatically improve the quality of a child's life. I once had a 17-year-old patient with ADHD tell me that on the first day that he took Ritalin, he had to pull over to the side of the road while driving home from school because he broke down in tears, saying to himself, "This must be what life is like for everyone." He felt he could finally "see" the world clearly and was so very sad that he had lived his whole life without the "benefit of glasses." Unfortunately, though, medication does not work for everyone, and it is not a panacea. For example, even though my patient could now see clearly, he still needed to learn strategies for organizing himself and for completing his homework. Understandably, his parents had always been reluctant to try medication, and it was not until he told them he was willing to try anything that they were willing to try it too. After the fact, he and his parents wished they had tried it sooner.

Although the information presented here on medication is only intended to get you started thinking about the process, it might be helpful to keep the following general guidelines in mind while you are thinking through this process:

- Medication should only be used as part of a comprehensive treatment because it is not a "cure all." Psychotherapy, counseling, and school support services often need to be used as well.
- Getting a thorough, comprehensive evaluation is essential before trying medication. Your doctor should be sure of the diagnosis before writing a prescription.
- Medication should be monitored closely by your child's physician. Sometimes this will be a pediatrician; other times it may be a child psychiatrist.
- Make sure all of your questions are answered before starting medication. Research has shown that the more comfortable people are with a medication or treatment approach, the more likely the treatment will work (perhaps because people will actually follow through with the treatment).
- Medication should not make your child a "zombie" or negatively change his personality. Medication should make your child seem more like him- or herself, not less, just without the troubling or burdensome symptoms he or she has.

- Medication does not always work, or sometimes it needs to be discontinued because of negative side effects that outweigh the benefits. Don't be afraid to try something else; it is common to try more than one medication before one works.

- Your child may not be the best judge of whether the medication is working, so it's important to get a report from teachers (in addition to your own judgment) to determine whether the medication is making a difference.

- Finally, medication is not for everyone, and if you have decided against it on the basis of all the available information, be confident of your decision. However, make sure your decision was not based on hearsay or unsubstantiated claims from the media. Make sure your decision is a rational one that is based on a close association with you, your doctor, and your child.

OCCUPATIONAL THERAPY

Sammy was a 6-year-old hyperactive boy who was having difficulty learning to write his letters. His teacher referred him for an evaluation because she was concerned about his overactivity, inattention, and problems completing schoolwork in first grade. I diagnosed Sammy with ADHD and recommended a number of treatments to address his problems with attention and impulsivity. However, my evaluation also indicated that Sammy was having significant problems with fine motor skills that were affecting his ability to write and to complete many school-related tasks, such as art projects, cutting, and drawing. I referred Sammy to an occupational therapist who evaluated his fine motor skills more specifically and recommended more specific treatment.

Occupational therapists treat both adults and children. In children, the focus is not on their "occupation" but on their ability to successfully develop life skills such as writing clearly, using tools

233

such as scissors, and feeding and dressing themselves. Occupational therapy is typically customized to the child's specific needs. Thus, treatment can include activities such as throwing a ball at a target, hitting a ball with a bat, or copying words written on a blackboard. In Sammy's case, the occupational therapist focused on developing his fine motor and visual motor skills so that he could more fully participate in the school curriculum, such as being able to write legibly and more fluently. She also helped his teacher modify classroom equipment, giving him a pencil with a larger grip and a more stable support base on which to do his work.

Children with many types of difficulties can benefit from occupational therapy, including children with

- learning disabilities,
- autism and pervasive developmental disorders,
- developmental delays,
- fine motor difficulties,
- problems with writing,
- low muscle tone and poor coordination, and
- brain injuries.

Occupational therapy can help improve many abilities, such as visual perception, writing, and fine motor skills. The goal of treatment is to make children more independent and improve normal development and performance. Occupational therapy can be done within or outside of the school environment, and if your child has a documented disability that requires occupational therapy, it is likely that he or she can receive services as part of his or her individual education plan. Occupational therapists work in hospitals, schools and in the community. They will use any combination of activities to strengthen muscles, increase movement, and improve coordination and balance. Within the schools, they will frequently modify school equipment and help the child participate as much as possible in school programs and activities.

PHYSICAL THERAPY

Physical therapy is frequently used to treat children who have been injured or who have a significant difficulty with gross motor skills. You may have used the services of a physical therapist after you have sustained an injury such as a broken bone or a torn ligament. Children who are treated with physical therapy usually have a developmental delay that makes it difficult for them to move in a way that is typical for their age. Physical therapy is often recommended for children with

- developmental delays,
- developmental disorders such as autism and pervasive developmental disorder,
- orthopedic disabilities,
- head trauma, and
- genetic disorders and birth defects that compromise gross motor skills such as Down syndrome or fragile X syndrome.

Physical therapy is usually customized to the needs of the child, but the treatment typically helps to build strength, improve movement, and strengthen skills needed to complete daily activities. This might include

- developmental activities such as crawling and walking;
- balance and coordination activities;
- activities to increase flexibility and strength;
- consulting with medication, psychiatric, and school personnel about goals for an individual education plan; and
- providing instructions for home exercise programs.

235

Overall, pediatric physical therapists specialize in the diagnosis and treatment of infants, children, and adolescents with a wide variety of developmental, congenital, or acquired disorders. Treatments focus on improving gross and fine motor skills, balance and coordination, and strength and endurance. Physical therapy usually treats children with developmental delays and problems that directly affect gross motor skills.

SPEECH AND LANGUAGE THERAPY

Speech and language therapists treat children who have language disorders (i.e., difficulty understanding or communicating ideas) or speech disorders (i.e., problems with the actual production of sounds). Speech disorders can include difficulty saying particular sounds or words; stuttering; problems with the pitch, volume, or quality of the voice; and problems with eating or swallowing. Language disorders can be either *expressive* or *receptive*. Expressive disorders refer to problems putting words together or difficulty using language in a socially appropriate way; receptive disorders refer to the difficulty understanding language. Children may be referred for speech and language disorders on the basis of the following:

- hearing impairments;
- cognitive deficits (i.e., problems with thinking skills that affect language);
- developmental delays;
- autism or pervasive developmental disorder;
- Asperger's syndrome (particularly as a result of problems with the social use of language skills);
- ADHD (as a result of problems in organizing one's thoughts); and
- learning disabilities, particularly language-based learning disabilities such as dyslexia and disorder of written expression.

My Child Was Just Evaluated and Found to Have Asperger's Syndrome. Her Language Skills Fell in the Superior Range. Why Did the Evaluator Recommend Speech and Language Therapy?

Good question! Speech and language therapy is frequently recommended for children with good language skills who have difficulty with *language pragmatics*. Pragmatics refers to social communication skills, such as sustaining eye contact, responding appropriately to a greeting, taking turns in conversation, or starting a conversation. Children with Asperger's syndrome often have relative weaknesses in these areas, and speech and language therapy can be quite effective in treating these difficulties.

How Do I Know I Am Getting a Qualified Occupational Therapist, Physical Therapist, or Speech and Language Therapist?

All three of these therapists require licensure to practice, so make sure your therapist is licensed by his or her board. In addition, you may want to ask a potential therapist the following questions:

- What is your area of specialty? How many children have you seen with that disorder?
- Are you licensed? How many years have you been practicing since licensure?
- Do you work with the school system and can you make recommendations to other professionals who are working with my child?
- Where did you receive your training?
- How will your treatment benefit my child?

Speech and language therapists work in hospitals, schools, and community clinics. If your child has a documented disability and receives services under his individual education plan, he may qualify for speech and language therapy. Speech therapy is typically customized to the child. For example, a child with autism may receive treatment focused on basic communication skills, such as improved eye contact and using words to communicate basic needs, whereas a child with dyslexia may receive treatment that includes phonological processing exercises and help with written expression.

CONCLUDING THOUGHTS

This chapter has provided only a glimpse into the most frequently suggested adjunct treatments for psychological, learning, and developmental issues. Keep in mind that treatment suggestions change over the course of development. For example, Sammy (described earlier) needed occupational therapy in first and second grade. This had the effect of remediating his handwriting problems, but by fourth grade his attentional problems had become impairing enough that he benefitted from medication. In eighth grade, he used the services of a speech and language therapist who specialized in the organization of language, including written language. Sammy had been having difficulty organizing his thoughts in a way that allowed him to write coherent papers. Speech and language therapy helped him learn strategies for organizing his thinking and expressive language, which in turn helped him to become a better writer. Throughout his elementary and middle school years, his parents consulted with a psychologist as needed for help with behavior management strategies while Sammy received as-needed psychotherapy from a psychologist who helped him process his emotions, learn more adaptive ways of behaving, and establish better coping skills in light of his diagnosis of ADHD.

ADDITIONAL RESOURCES

What follows is a list of books and websites of organizations that provide additional information on the topics presented in this book.

GENERAL INFORMATION

Books for Parents

Braaten, E., & Felopulos, G. (2004). *Straight talk about psychological testing for kids.* New York, NY: Guilford Press.
Faraone, S. V. (2003). *Straight talk about your child's mental health: What to do when something seems wrong.* New York, NY: Guilford Press.

Websites

http://www.aacap.org
    This website of the American Academy of Child and Adolescent Psychiatry provides information for families about mental illness and disorders, including where to get help and the latest information on psychiatric medications.

http://www.apa.org

The website of the American Psychological Association provides information for parents as well as referral information for parents seeking a psychologist in their area.

http://www.childadvocate.net

This website provides information to parents on mental health, educational, legal, and legislative issues.

http://www.dana.org

This website provides information about brain science and current brain research. The section "Brainy Kids Online" offers children, teens, and parents links to games and educational resources.

http://www.ffcmh.org

This is the website of the Federation of Families for Children's Mental Health.

http://www.mind.org.uk

"Mind" is a mental health organization based in England and Wales that provides links to information about mental health services in the United Kingdom as well as information and advice on mental health in children and adults.

http://www.miminc.org

The Madison Institute of Medicine provides an excellent website that offers information for parents on various psychological disorders including depression, obsessive–compulsive disorder, and bipolar disorder.

http://www.narsad.org

The National Alliance for Research on Schizophrenia and Depression provides up-to-date information about research on schizophrenia, depression, and bipolar disorder.

http://www.nimh.nih.gov

The website of this government agency, the National Institute of Mental Health, provides information about current research in mental health topics, clinical trials, and outreach programs.

http://www.our-kids.org

This website is "devoted to raising special kids with special needs."

ANXIETY AND OBSESSIVE–COMPULSIVE DISORDER

Books for Children and Adolescents

Harrar, G. (2004). *Not as crazy as I seem*. Boston, MA: Houghton Mifflin.

Sisemore, T. A. (2008). *I bet I won't fret: A workbook to help children with generalized anxiety disorder*. Oakland, CA: Instant Help Books.

Books for Parents

Chansky, T. (2001). *Freeing your child from obsessive-compulsive disorder*. New York, NY: Three Rivers Press.

Dacey, J., & Fiore, L. (2000). *Your anxious child*. San Francisco, CA: Jossey-Bass.

Fitzgibbons, L., & Pedrick, C. (2003). *Helping your child with OCD: A workbook for parents of children with obsessive-compulsive disorder*. Oakland, CA: New Harbinger.

Last, C. G. (2006). *Help for worried kids: How your child can conquer anxiety and fear*. New York, NY: Guilford Press.

March, J. S. (with Benton, C. M.). (2007). *Talking back to OCD: The program that helps kids and teens say "no way"— and parents say "way to go."* New York, NY: Guilford Press.

Rapee, R., Spence, S., Caham, V., & Wingnall, A. (2000). *Helping your anxious child: A step-by-step guide for parents.* Oakland, CA: New Harbinger.

Wagner, A. P. (2006). *What to do when your child has obsessive-compulsive disorder: Strategies and solutions.* Mobile, AL: Lighthouse Press.

Websites

http://www.adaa.org

The website of the Anxiety Disorders Association of America provides self-help tools, help with finding a therapist, and ways to cope with anxiety from preschool through college.

http://www.ocfoundation.org

The Obsessive–Compulsive Foundation educates parents of children with obsessive–compulsive disorder, maintains a list of providers, organizes support groups, and holds an annual conference.

ATTENTION-DEFICIT/HYPERACTIVITY DISORDER

Books for Kids and Teens

Nadeau, K. G., Dixon, E. B., & Beyl, C. (2004). *Learning to slow down and pay attention: A book for Kids about ADHD.* Washington, DC: Magination Press.

Walker, B. (2004). *The girls' guide to AD/HD: Don't lose this book!.* Bethesda, MD: Woodbine House.

Books for Parents

Barkley, R. A. (2000). *Taking charge of ADHD: The complete, authoritative guide for parents* (rev. ed.). New York, NY: Guilford Press.

Dendy, C. Z. (1995). *Teenagers with ADD: A parent's guide.* Bethesda, MD: Woodbine House.

Kolberg, J., & Nadeau, K. (2002). *ADD-friendly ways to organize your life.* New York, NY: Brunner-Routledge.

Monastra, V. J. (2005). *Parenting children with ADHD: 10 lessons that medicine cannot teach.* Washington, DC: American Psychological Association.

Nadeau, K., Littman, E., & Quinn, P. (2000). *Understanding girls with ADHD.* San Diego, CA: Advantage Books.

Zeigler Dendy, C. A. (2006). *Teenagers with ADD and ADHD: A parents' guide* (2nd ed.). Bethesda, MD: Woodbine House.

Websites

http://www.add.org

The website of the Attention Deficit Disorder Association provides information about ADHD, resources, support, and advocacy.

http://www.chadd.org

The website of the Children and Adults with Attention-Deficit/Hyperactivity Disorder provides information about resources for children and adults with ADHD as well as information about a yearly conference about ADHD and referrals to local practitioners who are knowledgeable about ADHD.

AUTISM, ASPERGER'S SYNDROME, AND PERVASIVE DEVELOPMENTAL DISORDERS

Books for Kids and Teens

Jackson, L. (2002). *Freaks, geeks, & Asperger's syndrome: A user's guide to adolescence.* London, England: Kingsley.

Tompkins, M. A., & Martinez, K. A. (2009). *My anxious mind: A teen's guide to managing anxiety and panic.* Washington, DC: Magination Press.

Books for Parents

Atwood, T. (2008). *The complete guide to Asperger's syndrome.* London, England: Kingsley.
Bashe, P. R., & Kirby, B. L. (2005). *The OASIS guide to Asperger syndrome: Advice, support, insight, and inspiration.* New York, NY: Crown.
Ozonoff, S., Dawson, G., & McPartland, J. (2002). *A parent's guide to Asperger syndrome and high-functioning autism.* New York, NY: Guilford Press.
Seroussi, K. (2002). *Unraveling the mystery of autism and pervasive developmental disorder.* New York, NY: Broadway Books.
Siegel, B. (2006). *Getting the best for your child with autism: An expert's guide to treatment.* New York, NY: Guilford Press.
Simpson, R.(with de Boer-Ott, S. R., Griswold, D., Myles, B. S., Byrd, S. E., Ganz, J., . . . Adams, L. G.). (2004). *Autism spectrum disorder: Inventions and treatments for children and youth.* Thousand Oaks, CA: Corwin Press.
Szatmari, P. (2004). *A mind apart: Understanding children with autism and Asperger syndrome.* New York, NY: Guilford Press.
Yapko, D. (2003). *Understanding autism spectrum disorders: Frequently asked questions.* London, England: Kingsley.

Websites

http://www.abaresources.com
This website provides information on applied behavior analysis for children with autism.

http://www.asperger.org

This website provides information about Asperger's syndrome, pervasive developmental disorder, and high-functioning autism.

http://www.aspergersyndrome.org

This website provides online Asperger's syndrome information and support for parents and students.

http://www.autism-society.org

The website of the Autism Society of America provides information about autism, Asperger's syndrome, and pervasive developmental disorder, including research, programs, and living with autism.

http://www.feat.org

This is the website of Families for Early Autism Treatment.

http://www.info.med.yale.edu/chldstdy/autism

The Yale Child Study Center provides this website, which answers questions about autism and reviews the latest research on autism spectrum disorders.

http://www.thearc.org

This website, operated by the Arc of the United States, is for individuals with developmental disabilities.

DISRUPTIVE BEHAVIOR DISORDERS

Books for Parents

Barkley, R., & Robin, A. (2008). *Your defiant teen: 10 steps to resolve conflict & rebuild your relationship.* New York, NY: Guilford Press.

Greene, R. (2005). *The explosive child.* New York, NY: Harper Collins.

Nichols, M. P. (2004). *Stop arguing with your kids: How to win the battle of wills by making your child feel heard.* New York, NY: Guilford Press.

Websites

http://www.ccbd.net
This website is sponsored by the Council for Children With Behavioral Disorders.

http://www.explosivekids.org
This is the website of the Foundation for Children With Behavioral Challenges.

EATING DISORDERS

Books for Teens

Nelson, T. (2008). *What's eating you: A workbook for teens with anorexia, bulimia, and other eating disorders.* Oakland, CA: Instant Help Books.
Wilhelm, S. (2006). *Feeling good about the way you look; A program for overcoming body image problems.* New York, NY: Guilford Press.

Books for Parents

Lock, J., & Grange, D. (2005). *Help your teenager beat an eating disorder.* New York, NY: Guilford Press.
Neumark-Sztainer, D. (2005). *"I'm like, so fat!": Helping your teen make healthy choices about eating and exercise in a weight-obsessed world.* New York, NY: Guilford Press.

Websites

http://www.anad.com

The website of the National Association of Anorexia Nervosa and Associated Eating Disorders provides information about eating disorders.

http://www.b-eat.co.uk

The website of the Beating Eating Disorders organization provides information, help, and support for individuals with eating disorders and their families.

LEARNING DISABILITIES

Books for Parents

Adelizzi, J. U. (2001). *Parenting children with learning disabilities.* Westport, CT: Bergin & Garvey Press.

Shaywitz, S. (2003). *Overcoming dyslexia: A new and complete science-based program for reading problems at any level.* New York, NY: Knopf.

Whitney, R. (2002). *Bridging the gap: Raising a child with nonverbal learning disorder.* New York, NY: Perigree Books.

Websites

http://www.advocacyinstitute.org

This website is operated by The Advocacy Institute and provides information about resources and services for children with learning disabilities.

http://www.cec.sped.org

This is the website of the Council for Exceptional Children.

http://www.ies.ed.gov/ncee/wwc/

This is the website of the What Works Clearinghouse and provides educators and parents with scientific evidence of what works in education.

http://www.interdys.org

The International Dyslexia Association operates this website.

http://www.ldanatl.org

The website of the Learning Disabilities Association of America offers information for parents and educators.

http://www.ldonline.org

This website provides information on learning disabilities and attention-deficity/hyperactivity disorder.

http://www.ncld.org

The website of the National Center for Learning Disabilities provides information about different types of learning disabilities as well as information about school services such as individual educational plans.

http://www.nldline.com

This is the website of Nonverbal Learning Disorder Online.

MEDICATION

Books for Parents

Brown, R. T., Carpenter, L.A., & Simerly, E. (2005). *Mental health medications for children: A primer.* New York, NY: Guilford Press.

Wilens, T. (2009). *Straight talk about psychiatric medications for kids.* New York, NY: Guilford.

Websites

http://www.parentsmedguide.org

This website of the American Psychiatric Organization provides information about medications for attention-deficit/hyperactivity disorder and depression in children.

MOOD DISORDERS

Books for Parents

Miklowitz, D. J. (2002). *The bipolar disorder survival guide: What you and your family need to know.* New York, NY: Guilford Press.

Papalos, D., & Papalos, J. (2006). *The bipolar child: The definitive and reassuring guide to childhood's most misunderstood disorder* (3rd ed.). New York, NY: Broadway Books.

Websites

http://www.bpkids.org

The website of the Child and Adolescent Bipolar Foundation provides information about bipolar disorder for parents, children, and adolescents.

http://www.depressionalliance.org

The Depression Alliance website (an organization based in the United Kingdom) provides information about depression, living with depression, treatments, and coping with depression.

http://www.depression.org

This is the website for the International Foundation for Research and Education on Depression.

http://www.familyaware.org

This website focuses on the effect of depression on the family.

SUBSTANCE ABUSE

Websites

http://www.addictionanswers.com

The website of the Addition Recovery Management System at Massachusetts General Hospital provides information for families, schools, and young adults about understanding addictions and recovery.

http://www.niaaa.nih.gov

The National Institute of Alcohol Abuse and Alcoholism website provides information regarding clinical trials, fact sheets on underage and college drinking, and recent research on alcohol abuse and treatment.

http://www.nida.nih.gov

This website is sponsored by the National Institute on Drug Abuse.

INDEX

ABOUT THE AUTHOR

Ellen B. Braaten, PhD, is an assistant professor at Harvard Medical School, the director of the Child Psychology Internship Training Program at Massachusetts General Hospital, and the director of the Learning and Emotional Assessment Program at Massachusetts General Hospital and Harvard Medical School. Dr. Braaten is a licensed child psychologist who specializes in pediatric neuropsychology and psychological testing. She has authored numerous scientific articles and chapters on children with attention-deficit/hyperactivity disorder, depression, anxiety, learning disabilities, and parenting. She is the coauthor of *Straight Talk About Psychological Testing for Kids* and the author of *The Child Clinician's Report-Writing Handbook*.